MW00562267

ROCKET FUEL ON A BUDGET

How to Get Healthy Without Going Broke

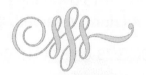

By

JOANNA RUSHTON

ROCKET FUEL ON A BUDGET

How to Get Healthy Without Going Broke

By

Joanna Rushton

www.energycoachinginstitute.com/rocket-fuel-on-a-budget/

PUBLISHED BY

Joanna Rushton

jo@energycoachinginstitute.com

Rocket Fuel on a Budget
Copyright © 2013 by Joanna Rushton
All rights reserved.

ISBN: 978-0-9874915-0-3

DISCLAIMER NOTICE

The information in this book is for informative purposes only and is the informed opinion of the author.

This book is designed to help you make better-informed decisions about your health, diet, and lifestyle choices. It is not intended nor should it be treated as a definitive guide on health and wellness, neither should it be regarded as medical or nutritional advice.

The author is not liable for your use of the ideas presented in this book; neither will she be held responsible for any health problem, loss, damage, claim or action that may result from the use of the information contained in this book.

Readers are advised to always consult their own health practitioners, doctors or physicians for professional advice on matters relating to their health and well-being.

Website

www.energycoachinginstitute.com/rocket-fuel-on-a-budget/

TABLE OF CONTENTS

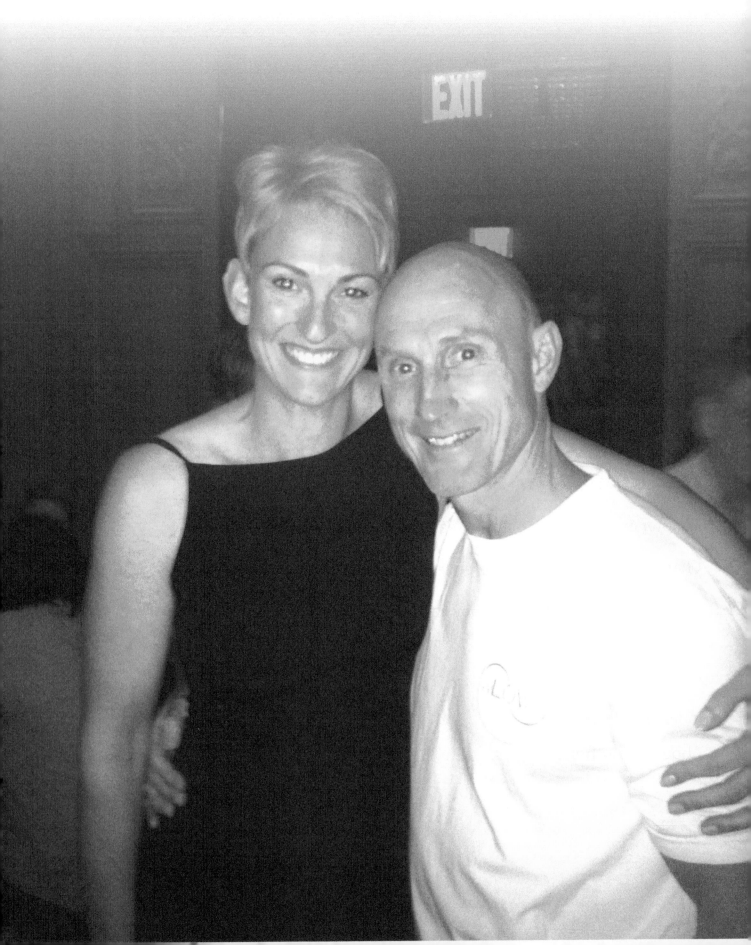

Rocket Fuel on a Budget

The book you are now reading is written by a beautiful, amazing, highly conscious and loving human being (who can see and read subtle energy fields). I have known Jo Rushton for over ten years, during which time she has studied my teachings extensively. Her level of commitment to herself and the world is truly exemplary. So exemplary, in fact, that I asked her to teach for the C.H.E.K Institute; an institute that teaches holistic health world-wide. She still does that beautifully today.

Jo is also an excellent chef. That I can attest to for sure!

Jo's knowledge comes from around the world - from different cultures and from intelligent people of diverse backgrounds. My testament to her wisdom is this: *the more simply you can express a complex message, the wiser you are.*

Thousands of hours of committed study and practice have been invested into the authenticity and creation of this book. Many have tried to say what Jo Rushton has shared here, but couldn't do it as elegantly as she has. 'If you want to become healthy, *you must first find a healthy teacher.*' You've succeeded in doing just that.

Now, all you need to do is follow her advice. The only side effects you will experience are likely to be:

More energy,
Better sex drive,
Better skin,
More favourable response to exercise,
Greater capacity to handle stress,
Optimal body shape,
and much more!

Love and chi,

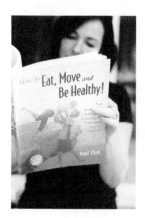

Paul Chek
Lover of Natural Life,
Holistic Health Practitioner,
Founder, C.H.E.K Institute and PPS Success Mastery Program

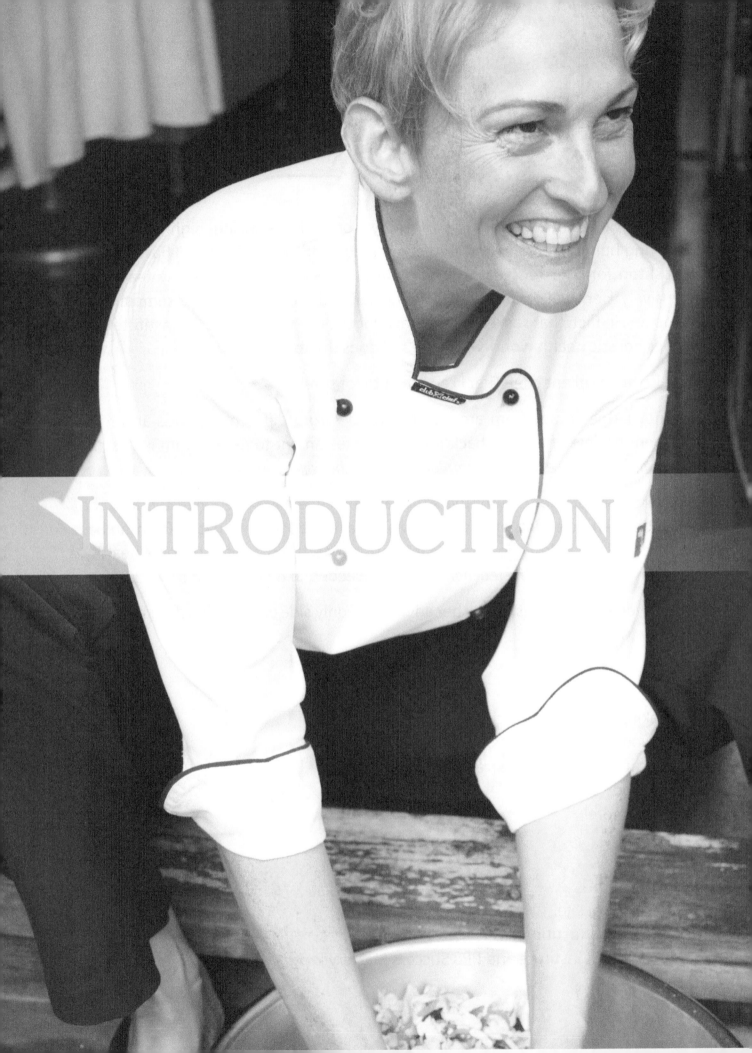

INTRODUCTION

Welcome to the Organic Chef Series, and thank you for purchasing my first book!

A message from me to you: Please scan this QR code with your iphone to view my you tube welcome message. <u>Welcome to Rocket Fuel on a Budget!</u>

The mere fact that you are reading this book indicates to me that you are already somewhat aware of the benefits of eating organically, and that you know that the choices you make affect your health, longevity and your environment. I also acknowledge that you have made the decision that you are worth the investment, which can sometimes be half the battle!

I have written this book in the hope that it will help you to avoid unnecessary financial stress when investing into yourself and your family's health. I want people to experience just how affordable and accessible eating organically can be. I don't want people to wait until they get sick, like I did, to realise that they could have prevented it had they known how to get healthy without going broke!

We are a family of four including two active, growing boys aged nine and eleven, both with healthy appetites, and we manage to eat organically 90% of the time.

My own story of recovery from chronic fatigue, IBS (irritable bowel syndrome) and leaky gut syndrome would not have been possible had I not chosen to take responsibility for the lifestyle choices that had contributed to the severe decline in my health. Ironically, I was a personal trainer at the time! I'm a great believer in the adage "we teach what we need to learn the most."

I bounced from Doctor to Specialist trying this treatment and that prescription which, at best, elevated the symptoms until, of course, I stopped them. Often, I would discover new symptoms that arose as a result of those treatments or medications. I eventually grew tired of just treating the symptoms and continuing to feel that the underlying cause was not being addressed.

It was at this time in my life and career that I was introduced to Paul Chek, a leading expert in holistic health, rehabilitation and sports-specific training. Paul is the founder of the C.H.E.K Institute in San Diego, California, and I am in deep gratitude to him for what I have learnt from him over the last 10 years. What I have come to realise is that no drug comes close to the effectiveness of nutrition, and there is absolutely no escaping the fact that the source and quality of the food we choose to fuel, nourish and heal ourselves with is the key foundation to achieving and maintaining good health and vitality.

My first career as a chef of twelve years afforded me the opportunity to travel and explore cultures and cuisines from Europe to South Africa to America, and now Australia, which has been my home for the last fourteen years. Little did I know, back then, that I was preparing myself with the skills that would later prove instrumental in the process of reclaiming my health and helping others to do the same.

My journey has been one step at a time. Slowly, I adopted all that I learned along the way into my lifestyle. As a result, I began to feel measurably better on all levels that pertain to my health and well-being. But there was something else; I also began to notice that I had an increasingly sizable food bill to cover each week which, if I wasn't careful, would start to create the sort of stress that could negatively impact my health, and I couldn't afford to go down that road again!

The purpose of this book is to provide you with real meal plans and recipes that will assist you in eating organic foods at very affordable prices.

The accompanying 21-day meal plan is designed for both the individual looking to make the first step towards improving their food and lifestyle choices, and the more experienced ones looking for structure with diversity and cost effectiveness.

I view prevention as a lifestyle, and I hope that this book provides you with the information, education and most importantly the inspiration you need to make sustainable choices towards a physically buoyant, financially balanced, and healthier you!

Warmly, Jo

CHAPTER 1

TOP 16 MISTAKES PEOPLE MAKE WHEN TRYING TO GET HEALTHY

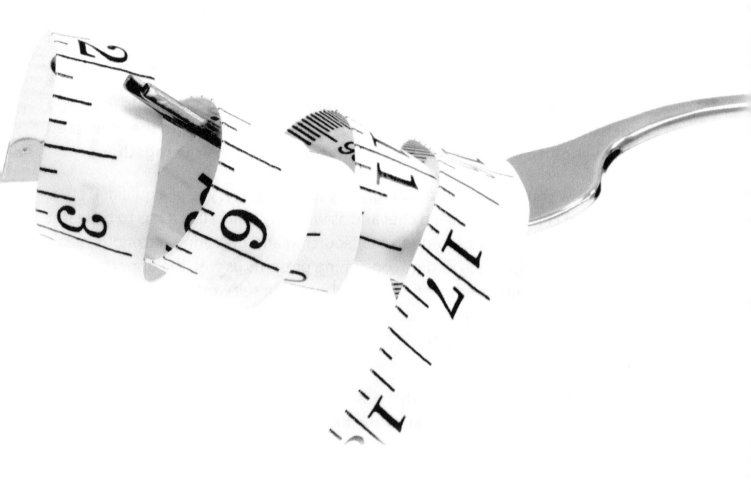

Over the past ten years of assisting other people in achieving physical, mental, emotional and spiritual health, I have come to observe a number of common assumptions, or call them 'beliefs', that hold true for the majority of the people I have coached on the subject of creating a healthier mind, body and lifestyle. The following are the top 16 misconceptions or beliefs people have when trying to get healthy:

1. The idea or belief that sourcing or preparing nutritious meals is all too expensive, too hard, takes too long, or is too complicated, and that you need to know how to cook before you can put something healthy together.

Okay right now you're probably thinking, "easy for you to say; you're a qualified chef." Yes, but I wasn't always a qualified chef and as with any skill in life, it has to be learnt and practiced. The idea or perception that sourcing and preparing nutritious meals is all too hard or complicated or time consuming presents us with the opportunity to see where we place our health, well-being and even our self worth on our priority list. The lower it sits as a priority, the more reasons we will give and the more resistance we will create to making the process feel difficult, hard and even painful. It is really far easier than you may think.

These misconceptions are largely what this book is about and I go into further details later on. However, in the first instance, we must think about the amount of money that we will save long term in avoiding medical and health bills when we eat foods that support and promote health and vitality as opposed to foods that diminish them.

2. Thinking exercise will forgive all sins.

This could be a book in its self! We have been fooled into thinking that weight loss is all about exercise alone. This misconception leads far too many people to rationalise their unhealthy eating habits. This myth can lead to over-training, poor recovery and burn-out. How many times have you justified junk food or decided how big a piece of cake you deserve for dessert based on how hard you worked out at the gym?

Exercise, when done correctly, can certainly assist to balance your biochemistry and metabolic processes, but it is the quality of the food you eat, the water you drink, and thoughts you think that determine the efficiency with which your body functions, far more than exercise. Research has shown that the balance is anything around 80% diet and 20% exercise when it comes to sustainable weight loss, health and longevity. Remember, your workouts are only as good as the food you fuel your workouts with. If you want to train effectively and efficiently and see remarkable results for doing so, then what you choose to do when you're not in the gym is of equal importance. Exercise is an ADJUNCT to a healthy eating plan; NOT a substitute.

3. Believing that cardio vascular exercise is the best way to get fit and lose weight.

This is another exercise myth! Repetitive movement such as running or aerobics can lead to muscular imbalances and related injuries. Contrary to popular belief, weight resistant or anabolic exercises are more effective at burning fat than aerobic or cardiovascular exercises. It is well known that muscle weighs more than fat, and that anaerobic exercise, like resistant weight training, increases your muscle mass which in turn increases your resting metabolic rate, which results in weight loss.

Resistant weight training, when performed correctly, lowers cortisol levels (the body's stress hormone) and increases your repair, growth, reproductive and anti-ageing hormones. Excessive aerobic exercise for prolonged periods however increases cortisol while decreasing your repair, growth, reproductive and anti-ageing hormones. This increases the overall stress levels of the body, which further inhibits the body's ability to lose fat, and promotes muscle loss and tone. Women especially become even more efficient at holding fluid and storing fat when they are stressed!

4. Believing that you have to count or cut calories to lose weight

The skipping of any meal or not eating enough of the right foods immediately sends the body into survival mode. This stress response elevates your blood sugar (insulin) levels. With repeated or prolonged periods of unsustainable dieting, the body switches into famine mode and stores any energy whenever given. Deborah Woodhouse in her book *Outsmarting the Female Fat Cell* showed women to have more fat-storing enzymes than men. She also showed how missing just one meal increases the release of lipogenic (fat-storing) enzymes that subsequently decreases the desired lipolytic (fat-burning) enzymes. This is far more prevalent in women than in men. If you eat and exercise correctly, you shouldn't need to over or under eat.

5. The ALL or NOTHING attitude

Changing lifestyle behaviours and forming new habits takes time and energy. By the time most people realise that something has to change, they are already feeling exhausted and depleted of energy. Trying to change everything all at once can become too overwhelming and feel too hard, at which point most people just give up. Always prioritise and choose the one thing that will give you the most return for your efforts. This means you will have increasingly more energy to integrate the next prioritised change. One step at a time is the key.

6. Failing to plan = planning to fail

As with the ALL or NOTHING attitude, good intentions alone aren't enough to keep us adherent to a new habit. Until the new choices are fully integrated into your everyday life, it's very likely that you will return to your old habits, especially when you feel inconvenienced or stressed out. Creating a structured plan will help minimise self-sabotage or the convenience and comfort of old ways.

7. Relying on discipline alone to reach your goals

Of course discipline is an essential ingredient, however, unless you have a strong enough motive, chances are discipline alone won't be enough. Make sure that the changes you need to make can be correlated into supporting your over-arching dream or purpose in life. Then when you break down the BIG dream into smaller goals, make sure they appeal to the mind AND the heart. The SMART analogy, as it stands, is very appealing to the left side of the brain that looks for structure, planning and measurable outcomes. However when you set goals that also speak to your heart and the right side of your brain, you will stand a far greater chance of adhering to and achieving your goals. Turn SMART goals into HEART goals!

Brain	Heart
Specific	**S**ustainable
Measurable	**M**eaningful
Achievable	**A**ligned to your dream
Realistic	**R**ewarding
Timely	**T**angible

8. Believing that foods labelled "natural" or "organic" determine whether the food is truly healthy

Here's where we fall pray to the Food Industry and their marketing jargon. They use buzzwords they think will sell their products. Terms like "natural" or "organic" are useless if the product in question is loaded with sugar (organic or not), or if the product contains highly processed ingredients and/ additives. Labelling laws designed to 'protect the consumer' are questionable at best. Learn to read the fine print in the actual nutritional analysis and understand the ingredients listed. The ingredients are usually listed in order of what the product constitutes, from the most to the least. Remember, it is only organic if there is a stamp certifying it to be organic. Another good tip is; if the ingredients weren't around when your great grandma was alive, chances are your liver won't like it!

Here are some examples of what I mean by organic products trying to pass themselves off as healthy under the umbrella of "organic", when the sugar content and processed nature, in my opinion, undermines the intention for what organic truly stands for.

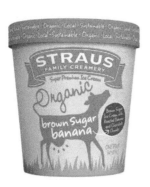 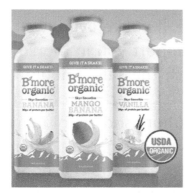 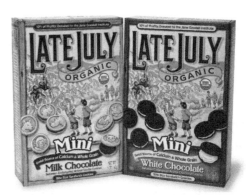

9. Putting your trust into Dieticians, Nutritionists, Doctors and the media for nutritional information.

Remember, most 'mainstream' sources for nutritional information or advice has an inherent agenda, whether obvious or not. Any mainstream source providing 'education' on how or what you need in order to be healthy is most probably, directly or indirectly, furthering the financial interests of various multinational corporations, mainstream medicine and/ pharmaceutical companies. This is not conspiracy, paranoia or cynicism; it is reality.

There is considerable reason to be cautious. Medical doctors, although often well meaning, may be the single most unqualified people to offer nutritional recommendations. Their education in nutrition totals an average of five hours over five years and is carefully cultivated by medical schools entirely toward the promotion of pharmaceutical interests. Is it really 'health' that is studied in medical schools, or is it rather 'diseases and their treatments with the use of drugs, surgery and other medical procedures'?

I am not suggesting that you ignore the advices of your healthcare provider, however I would rather you be very cautious, do your homework and seek second or multiple opinions wherever possible. No one will ever care more about your health than you.

Mainstream dieticians and nutritionists generally use a working model based on the unfounded and unscientific USDA Food Pyramid. The pharmaceutical companies and food corporations fund the vast majority of research used to support 'mainstream' nutritional advice and, till date, the evidence that it works is far from compelling.

Not surprisingly, the media, on nearly all fronts, remain loyal to the interests of their advertisers - the food corporations and pharmaceutical industries. They cannot afford to be objective or tell the truth when millions of their advertising revenues are dependent on funding from fast foods, processed foods and drug companies.

10. Once in a while can't hurt... CAN IT?

Generally, I believe in the 80/20 rule. If you're living well 80% of the time, your body's constitution of health will support you in the 20% exception. However, there are certain non-foods of which the safe amount to consume are ZERO. These foods I'm referring to are trans-fats used for cooking french-fries, chips and many confectionery products. MSG (monosodium glutamate), GMO (genetically modified organism) and processed white sugar are other non-foods that, in my opinion, should never enter the 20% exception. If good health really matters to you, then the less you compromise yours, the better for you. Interestingly, my personal experience and that of my clients is that the 80% will eventually show you the pain associated with the 20% exception. As a person gets healthier and healthier, their awareness increases along with the realisation that the 20% exception just isn't worth the compromise.

11. Believing in the Food Pyramid recommendations

Just how safe or effective are governments' guidelines and The Food Pyramid for building and supporting optimal health? Take a look at the escalating rate of obesity, diabetes, heart disease, alcoholism and any other degenerative illness you can think of in the community. Look at life expectancy. Consider also what now constitutes as 'food' under our governments' guidelines and you would have no choice but to agree that they are questionable at best. The same government that once endorsed the safety of trans-fats and promoted them as a saturated fat alternative, some 10 years later, revoked its endorsement and made it illegal in parts of the United States, whilst other countries like Russia have banned the import of US GMO corn from *Monsanto Co.*

Turn 'The Food Pyramid' upside down and you would straight away have made improvements. A food pyramid that has proved to represent a far more comprehensive guide to foods and their consumption is David Getoff's food pyramid, simply Google 'David Getoff food pyramid' and take a look at the differences!

12. Jane is 'thin', she MUST be healthy. Think again.

WARNING: DANGER AHEAD! Thinking that being slim or using your weight as a benchmark for good health can lead you sooner or later into some serious problems. Although it's always better not to be overweight, looking good on the outside by no way means everything is working right on the inside. 98% of all disease begins in the gut. It is entirely possible to be slim AND diabetic. It is entirely possible to be slim AND suffer a heart attack or stroke. It is entirely possible to be slim AND get cancer, or any other disease. Using the superficial cultural image of being slim as your benchmark to being healthy can have devastating consequences on your health. Diet programs designed to help you lose weight typically focus on 'low calories' to the exclusion of quality-sourced and nutritionally dense foods.

13. Thinking that taking a multi-vitamin or supplement will make up for less healthy habits.

Keep in mind that vitamins and supplement companies are profit-oriented organisations. Many would like you to believe that you can make up for a lack of nutrients in your diet by just taking their "One a Day" multi-vitamin. There is no such thing! Supplements are just that - supplements. They can be a useful addition to an already healthy diet and can bridge the gap when an individual's constitution of health is so low that their ability to break down, digest and absorb food is significantly impaired. They, however, can never E-V-E-R be a substitute.

One of the key roles of a secondary nutrient is to break down and make available to the body the nutrients held within the whole food you eat. If you're eating rubbish food and supplementing with a multi-vitamin, you're just helping the body to breakdown and absorb the rubbish you are eating!

Please remember that all vitamins, supplements and even drugs originate from plants in nature. The key difference with synthetic vitamins is that they are not in the complete form as they are found in nature, and therefore will never have the same therapeutic effect on the body as they would when eating foods that contain the secondary nutrients in its complete and complex form. If you need to supplement with vitamins, make sure they are whole food supplements, and not synthetic, and that you do so under the guidance of a qualified health practitioner; one that knows how to work with vitamins, minerals and supplements.

14. Believing that you are destined for the same health problems that plagued your family.

The science of Epigenetics is now showing us that our nutrition, environment and even our thoughts affect the future expression of our genes. Our genes are no longer seen as the pre-determining factor over the future of our health. Don't believe, just because your mother or grandmother suffered high blood pressure or heart attacks, or that because there are many overweight people in your family, that you will automatically follow suit. We now KNOW we have the ability to influence our genes and unlock the full potential of our individual genetic expression whilst suppressing our genetic weaknesses. In the book *Biology of Belief,* Bruce Lipton, an American developmental biologist who is well-known for promoting the idea that genes and DNA can be manipulated by a person's beliefs, describes how we can change our DNA by changing the way we process our thoughts and experiences.

Knowing that ALL our choices affect how our genes express themselves and that our genetic pool no longer has to be a death sentence is very empowering. To know that we can directly influence and change our own genetic make up and that of our offspring, shows that we can't hide behind victim mentality anymore; that we can change the quality of our health on all levels of our being. I'm healthier now in my 40s than I was in my 30s because I have been living and abiding by these principles consciously and consistently for the last five years. And you can too!

15. Buying into the idea that Soy products are a healthy alternative to dairy or animal protein

Over the last twenty years, soy products have been given as much good hype as saturated fats have been given a bad rap. Here are some true and false facts regarding soy. Corn and soy are two of the largest produced crops of GMO foods today.

Myth: Use of soy as a food dates back many thousands of years.

Truth: Soy was first used as a food during the late Chou dynasty (1134 - 246 BC), only after the Chinese learned to ferment soy beans to make foods like *tempeh, natto* and *tamari*.

Myth: Asians consume large amounts of soy foods.

Truth: Average consumption of soy foods in Japan and China is 10 grams (about 2 teaspoons) per day. Asians consume soy foods in small amounts as a condiment, and not as a replacement for animal foods.

Myth: Modern soy foods confer the same health benefits as traditionally fermented soy foods.

Truth: Most modern soy foods are not fermented to neutralize toxins in soybeans, and are processed in ways that denature proteins and increase the levels of carcinogens.

Myth: Soy foods provide complete protein.

Truth: Like all legumes, soy beans are deficient in sulfur-containing amino acids Methionine and Cystine. In addition, modern processing denatures fragile lysine.

Myth: Fermented soy foods can provide Vitamin B12 in vegetarian diets.

Truth: The compound that resembles Vitamin B12 in soy cannot be used by the human body; in fact, soy foods cause the body to require more B12

Myth: Soy formula is safe for infants.

Truth: Soy foods contain trypsin inhibitors that inhibit protein digestion and affect pancreatic functions. In test animals, diets high in trypsin inhibitors led to stunted growth and pancreatic disorders. Soy foods increase the body's requirement for Vitamin D, needed for strong bones and normal growth. Phytic acid in soy foods results in reduced bio-availability of iron and zinc which are required for the health and development of the brain and nervous system. Soy also lacks cholesterol, likewise essential for the development of the brain and nervous system. Mega doses of phytoestrogens in soy formula have been implicated in the current trend toward increasingly premature sexual development in girls and delayed or retarded sexual development in boys.

Myth: Soy foods can prevent osteoporosis.

Truth: Soy foods can cause deficiencies in calcium and Vitamin D (both needed for healthy bones). Calcium from bone broths, Vitamin D from seafood, lard and organ meats prevent osteoporosis in Asian countries - not soy foods.

Myth: Modern soy foods protect against many types of cancer.

Truth: A British government report concluded that there is little evidence that soy foods protect against breast cancer or any other forms of cancer. In fact, soy foods may result in an increased risk of cancer.

Myth: Soy foods protect against heart disease.

Truth: In some people, consumption of soy foods will lower cholesterol, but there is no evidence that lowering cholesterol reduces one's risk of having heart disease.

Myth: Soy estrogens (isoflavones) are good for you.

Truth: Soy isoflavones are phyto-endocrine disrupters. At dietary levels, they can prevent ovulation and stimulate the growth of cancer cells. Eating as little as 30 grams (about 4 tablespoons) of soy per day can result in hypothyroidism with symptoms of lethargy, constipation, weight gain and fatigue.

Myth: Soy foods are safe and beneficial for women to use in their postmenopausal years.

Truth: Soy foods can stimulate the growth of estrogen-dependent tumours and cause thyroid problems. Low thyroid function is associated with difficulties in menopause.

Myth: Phytoestrogens in soy foods can enhance mental ability.

Truth: A recent study found that women with the highest levels of estrogen in their blood had the lowest levels of cognitive function; In Japanese-Americans, tofu consumption in mid-life is associated with the occurrence of Alzheimer's disease in later life.

Myth: Soy isoflavones and soy protein isolate have GRAS (Generally Recognized as Safe) status.

Truth: Archer Daniels Midland (ADM) recently withdrew its application to the FDA for GRAS status for soy isoflavones following an outpouring of protest from the scientific community. The FDA never approved GRAS status for soy protein isolate because of concern regarding the presence of toxins and carcinogens in processed soy.

Myth: Soy foods are good for your sex life.

Truth: Numerous animal studies show that soy foods cause infertility in animals. Soy consumption enhances hair growth in middle-aged men, indicating lowered testosterone levels. Japanese housewives feed tofu to their husbands frequently when they want to reduce his virility.

Myth: Soy beans are good for the environment.

Truth: Most soy beans grown in the US are genetically engineered to allow farmers to use large amounts of herbicides.

Myth: Soy beans are good for developing nations.

Truth: In third world countries, soybeans replace traditional crops to transfer the burden of processing from the local population to multinational corporations.

© 1999 Weston A. Price Foundation. All Rights Reserved.

16. Believing that you have to eat 'low fat' and forego dietary cholesterol to enjoy good health

The mainstream consensus is that eating 'low fat' and 'low cholesterol' products is good for our health and lowers the risk of heart disease. This is one of the BIGGEST myths in the health and fitness industry. Our genetic lineage is proof that we are designed to consume a diet rich in animal food sources and natural fats, together with a variety of fibrous plant matter. Dr. Weston A Price's comprehensive scientific global study of over 10 years in the 1920s and 30s proved this theory. In his book *Nutrition and Physical Degeneration*, he documents the study of up to 16 different primitive cultures across 14 countries; from villages in Switzerland, to Gaelic communities in the Outer Hebrides, to Eskimos and Indians of North America, Melanesian and Polynesian South Sea Islanders, African tribes, Australian Aborigines, New Zealand Maori and the Indians of South America. He was unable to find one culture that was strictly 100% vegetarian. Being a vegetarian himself this was both a surprise and possibly a disappointment to him, as he documented that the cultures that had less access to animal products in their diets were notably less vital in their constitution of health.

Vegetarianism and veganism are modern day ideas based more on political ideological principles than the foundations that underpin the nutrition needed for healthy human physiology.

Animal-sourced foods are however only as healthy as their source. No one should be eating pesticide-laden, or hormone and antibiotic-treated animals. Due to consumer demand, it is easy to find healthy, ethically and naturally raised organic animal food sources that we have been physiologically adapted to eating, for at least the last 2.6 million years.

Butter and other clean and natural sources of saturated fat are not a sin! They are the essential nutrient that when consumed in balance for your individual needs deliver adequate amounts of dietary cholesterol and other vital nutrients to the body. Cholesterol is vital for the production of all steroid hormones such as cortisol, the body's stress hormone, as well as the repair, growth, reproductive and anti-ageing hormones. When you truly understand the vital role that cholesterol plays in the body, you realise that by not consuming adequate amounts of dietary cholesterol, you force your body to function solely on making its own, which puts severe and

11

unnecessary additional stress on the body that can actually lead to increased blood cholesterol levels.

Some excellent resources on the subject are *The Great Cholesterol Con* by Dr Malcolm Kendrick, *Primal Mind, Primal Body* by Nora Gedgaudas and the work of Uffe Ravnskov MD PhD.

> *"He who does not know food; how can he understand the disease of man?"*
> *- Hippocrates, the father of medicine.*
> *(460-c. 370B.C)*

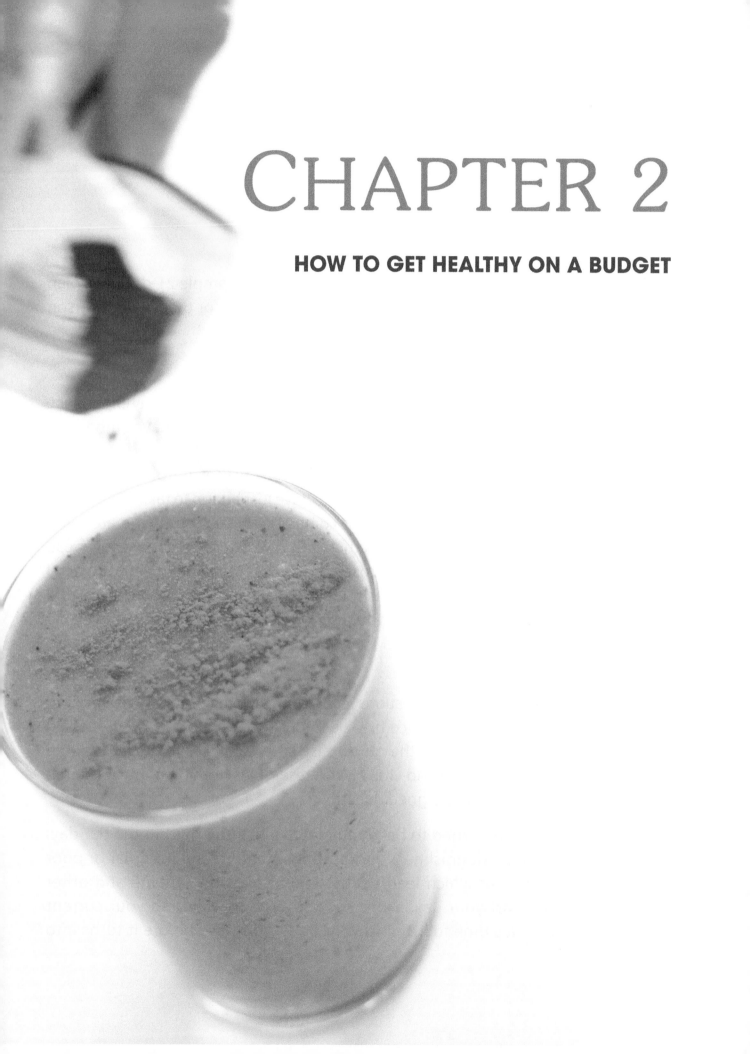

CHAPTER 2

HOW TO GET HEALTHY ON A BUDGET

The purpose of this book is to provide the reader with a sample 21-day meal plan that is both healthy and affordable, and that is suitable for the average person or family.

Why 21 days?

Well, research says it takes a minimum of 21 days to form a new habit. In my experience it often takes longer, however try the 21 days and you will certainly have embedded some great new eating habits. Based on an average spend of $17.00 per day for the single adult person, this equates to an average of $119 a week for breakfast, lunch and dinner. I wanted to appeal to both those who have just begun to take more notice and care about what they eat and where it comes from, and those who are more experienced and are still looking for structure with diversity and cost effectiveness. Eating organically has such a stigma of cost and expense surrounding it, yet when I work with clients and families to educate them on qualifying their food choices and their sources, about half of what they would spend their money on (non-perishable processed items) becomes redundant. There's your first saving that goes back into buying nutrient-rich organic foods.

You will notice that the meal suggestions, especially for breakfast, are designed to replace the modern day convenience breakfast foods that are based on processed carbohydrates that, whilst having the quick, easy and ready to eat appeal, lack the vital nutrients that build health and vitality, and resembles nothing of the food that we have evolved from or are designed to eat.

These meal plans are designed to help you create a healthy rhythm to your day; a rhythm that combats sluggishness, indigestion, bloating and irregular or poor bowel movements all of which lead to the dependency on caffeine and other stimulants to kick start your day. If this sounds all too familiar to your current daily rhythms, then it's time to listen to your body's dis-ease before it turns into a disease.

An open mind and a willingness to confront the norm will help you make more conscious meal choices that nourish your body as well as fuel it with the energy you want and deserve.

This meal plan will appeal to both those who are inspired to learn about making healthier food choices, and those who already are. Therefore, there's something here for everyone. The key objectives are:

➤ To get people eating a healthy breakfast option as opposed to no breakfast at all.

➤ To offer an easy to follow meal plan that provides structure to a busy working week.

➤ To increase the intake of freshly sourced and prepared produce.

➤ To ensure each meal consists of quality-sourced and unprocessed carbohydrate, protein and fat.

➤ To introduce slow cooking as a cooking method that saves money and offers ease, simplicity and time efficiency.

➤ To utilize the cook-once-eat-twice philosophy to reduce the use of processed and convenience foods, take out, meal replacements, protein shakes and reliance on supplements.

➤ To build basic skills and confidence in the kitchen.

➤ To introduce the value of fermented and cultured foods.

➤ To give you the skill and knowledge to use food as your medicine.

➤ To support your body's natural healing capabilities.

Below is a basic readiness questionnaire that will help you decide if you're ready for this 21-day challenge!

Meal plan readiness questionnaire

If you answer 'yes' to 4 or more of the statements in the questionnaire, then I recommend you start with this 21-day meal plan. Focus on making breakfast your priority and taking dinner leftovers to work for your lunch. You can progress to following the whole meal plan in your own time.

If you answered 'no' to 4 or more of the statements in the questionnaire, then you are ready to follow the meal plan as it is. You can also add in your own variations and product alternatives. You may discover that you have less of a need to rely on leftovers, if you are already in the habit of being organised in preparing your meals ahead of time.

Q 1: I leave home without eating breakfast more than once a week? Yes / No.

Q 2: I buy take-outs or ready-made meals, for home/office use more than twice per week? Yes / No.

Q 3: I shop for fresh produce less than 3 times per week? Yes / No.

Q 4: I eat out more than twice per week? Yes / No.

Q 5: I buy lunch at work more than twice per week? Yes / No.

Q 6: I buy non-organic produce more than organic produce? Yes / No.

Q 7: I use a microwave? Yes / No.

Q 8: I am not very confident in the kitchen when preparing and cooking food, and I find most recipes overwhelming? Yes / No.

PLANNING AHEAD

All the planning has quite literally been done for you. Once you have chosen your meal plan, it is as simple as making your shopping list for your chosen meal plan based on the single person, couple or family of four. Use the resource lists in *Chapter 7* and the tips offered in *Chapter 5*. Read Jo's tips where required and trust in yourself and the process, and have fun!

PANTRY ESSENTIALS

Every home larder or pantry should have the following fundamentals always on hand. This will help you to create a tasty and healthy meal in minutes even if you only came home with nothing but chicken and broccoli!

Organic eggs

Organic coconut oil

Organic tinned coconut milk

Organic Olive Oil

Organic Balsamic vinegar

Organic Tamari soy sauce

Organic raw honey

Organic chicken, beef or vegetable stock (fresh is best but minimally processed powder or carton is useful to have on hand)

Organic tinned chopped tomatoes

Organic tinned legumes, chickpeas, kidney beans, cannellini beans, etc

Organic tomato paste

Celtic or Himalayan sea salt

Selection of organic dried fruit e.g. raisins, dates, apricots, etc

Selection of organic nuts

Black pepper

A variety of mixed herbs and spices

Other basic items that are always handy to have at hand, have a longer shelf life, can be stored in a cool dry space and don't need refrigeration are root vegetables including:

Onions

Potatoes

Carrots

Fresh garlic & ginger

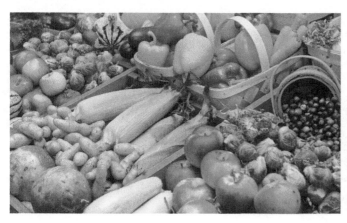 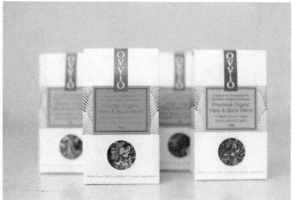

"If we could give every individual the right amount of nourishment and exercise - not too little, not too much - we would have the safest way to health."
- Hippocrates, the father of medicine
(406-c. 370 B.C)

CHAPTER 3

21 DAY MEAL PLAN AND RECIPES

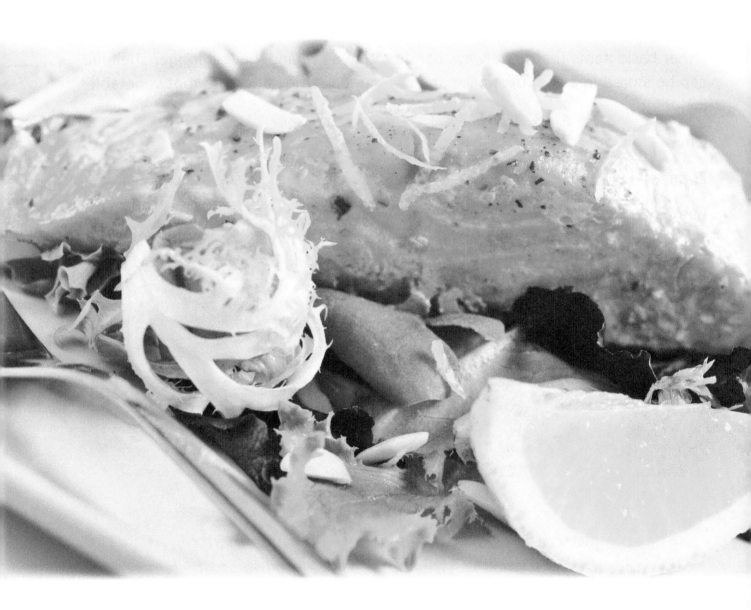

MEAL PLAN

Mon 1:

BREAKFAST: Fresh coconut & blueberry power smoothie.

LUNCH: Leftovers from Sunday's dinner.

SNACKS: Pear with a handful of raw almonds.

DINNER: Slow-cooked lemon & thyme, chicken Maryland's with mixed steamed vegetables.

Tue 2:

BREAKFAST: Sliced tomato & avocado, cracked pepper on toasted Sourdough bread.

LUNCH: Tandoori grilled chicken thigh & salad.

SNACKS: Chicken liver pate with sliced apple.

DINNER: Lamb Moussaka & salad.

Wed 3:

BREAKFAST: Stewed fruit compote with cultured yoghurt & young coconut flesh.

LUNCH: Leftovers from Tuesday's dinner.

SNACKS: Guacamole & corn chips.

DINNER: Aromatic coconut Fish Curry.

Thu 4:

BREAKFAST: Quark cheese with sliced tomato, cracked pepper on Rye sourdough.

LUNCH: Roasted vegetable and basil frittata and salad.

SNACKS: Apple with a handful of raw macadamia nuts.

DINNER: Thai Chicken Larb and crispy lettuce.

Fri 5:

BREAKFAST: Fresh coconut & banana power smoothie.

LUNCH: Leftovers from Thursday's dinner.

SNACKS: Baba Ghanouj with cucumber sticks.

DINNER: Poached Barramundi with ginger and lemon grass.

Sat 6:

BREAKFAST: Poached eggs & bacon with steamed asparagus & cherry tomatoes.

LUNCH: Prawn and avocado salad with toasted coconut.

SNACKS: Mixed nut spread with sliced carrots.

DINNER: Homemade kangaroo burgers with a pear and Persian goats cheese salad.

Sun 7:

BREAKFAST: Apple & cinnamon buckwheat pancakes with cultured yoghurt & a drizzle of maple syrup.

LUNCH: Salmon cutlet with a green apple salad.

SNACKS: Full fat quark cheese with celery sticks.

DINNER: Mexican style stuffed Peppers.

Mon 8:

BREAKFAST: Quinoa porridge with nuts, cultured yoghurt and a drizzle of honey.

LUNCH: Leftovers from Sunday's dinner.

SNACKS: Banana with a handful of crispy pecans.

DINNER: Slow-cooked Persian chicken.

Tue 9:

BREAKFAST: Fresh coconut & mixed berry power smoothie.

LUNCH: Grilled sausages with steamed vegetables.

SNACKS: Hard-boiled egg, carrot sticks.

DINNER: Slow-cooked spiced pork with apple and fennel.

Wed 10:

BREAKFAST: Smoked salmon avocado, cracked pepper on toasted Sourdough.

LUNCH: Leftovers from Tuesday's dinner.

SNACKS: Salsa & corn chips.

DINNER: Jo's favourite fish pie.

Thu 11:

BREAKFAST: Homemade raw cottage cheese & mixed herbs, tomato, cracked pepper on Rye sourdough.

LUNCH: Tinned sardines or tuna with salad.

SNACKS: Apple with a handful of raw macadamia nuts.

DINNER: Beef cheeks with onion thyme & mushrooms.

Fri 12:

BREAKFAST: Soft-boiled eggs topped with butter and fresh parsley & steamed green beans.

LUNCH: Leftovers from Thursday's dinner.

SNACKS: Raw date & nut slice.

DINNER: Chicken & vegetable curry.

Sat 13:

BREAKFAST: Gravlax salmon thimble of scramble eggs and chives.

LUNCH: Chicken burgers and salad.

SNACKS: Full fat quark cheese with celery sticks.

DINNER: Poached snapper with leek and fennel.

Sun 14:

BREAKFAST: Grilled lamb sausages with a medley of sautéed tomatoes, mushrooms & spinach.

LUNCH: Grilled calamari and salad.

SNACKS: Leftover lamb sausage with an apple.

DINNER: Braised duck with figs, honey and vinegar.

Mon 15:

BREAKFAST: Stewed fruit compote with cultured yoghurt & young coconut flesh.

LUNCH: Leftovers from Sunday's dinner.

SNACKS: Guacamole & carrot sticks.

DINNER: Poached lemon myrtle chicken with braised vegetables.

Tue 16:

BREAKFAST: Quark cheese with sliced tomato, cracked pepper on Rye sourdough.

LUNCH: Stir-fried chicken, broccoli ginger, shallots and cashews.

SNACKS: Baba Ghanouj with cucumber sticks.

DINNER: Slow-roasted shoulder of lamb with roasted vegetables.

Wed 17:

BREAKFAST: Roasted Vegetable and basil frittata.

LUNCH: Leftovers from Tuesday's dinner.

SNACKS: Slice of frittata.

DINNER: Poached salmon with fresh ginger, lemongrass and mint.

Thu 18:

BREAKFAST: Fresh coconut & mix berry power smoothie.

LUNCH: Tinned sardines or tuna with salad.

SNACKS: Fresh coconut & cinnamon smoothie.

DINNER: Chicken moussaka & salad.

Fri 19:

BREAKFAST: Sliced tomato & avocado, cracked pepper on toasted Sourdough bread.

LUNCH: Leftovers from Thursday's dinner.

SNACKS: Chicken liver pate with sliced apple.

DINNER: Pork stir-fried with fresh ginger, garlic and chilli.

Sat 20:

BREAKFAST: Baked eggs with Tuscan herbs & shaved leg of ham.

LUNCH: Thai beef salad.

SNACKS: Apple with a handful of raw macadamia nuts.

DINNER: Slow-cooked lamb Kashmir.

Sun 21:

BREAKFAST: Salmon & dill fish cakes topped with a fried egg.

LUNCH: Poached coconut chicken with a tropical salsa.

SNACKS: Tahini and celery sticks.

DINNER: Tandoori grilled chicken thigh & salad.

If you lack time and you're looking for a healthy and fast breakfast choice, then leftovers from dinner win hands down every time.

Recipes
FOR 21-DAY
Meal Plan

BREAKFASTS

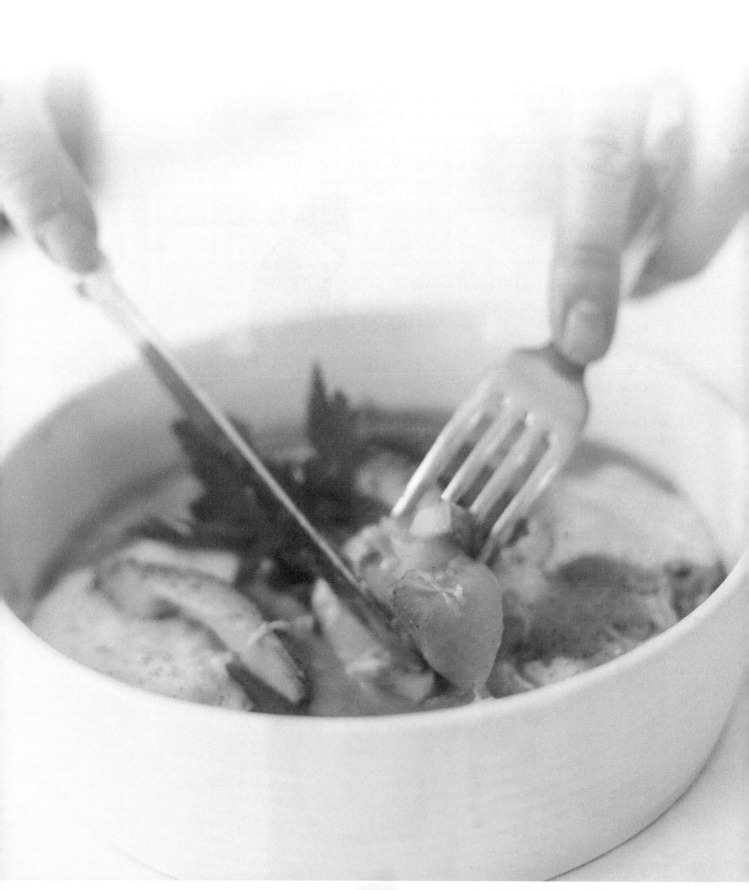

fresh coconut power smoothie

Serves two @ $3.20 per serve

2 raw organic eggs	1 tbsp. of coconut oil
The water and flesh of 1 Thai drinking fresh coconut	1 tsp. of cinnamon
	A few drops of pure vanilla extract o[...] powder.

Choose from the following smoothie elixir combinations:

1. Mixed berry & vanilla: ½ cup of frozen or fresh berries and ¼ tsp. of vanilla powder.

2. Banana & nutmeg: add ¼ tsp. of nutmeg.

3. Ginger & mango: 1 tsp. of fresh grated ginger and ½ cup of fresh or frozen mango.

4. Pineapple & honey: ½ cup of pineapple & ½ tsp. of honey.

5. Banana, mango, cashews & ginger: ½ cup of banana, ½ cup of mango, 1 tbsp. of cashews and 1 tsp. of grated ginger.

6. Almonds, banana, dates: 1 tsp. of almonds, ½ cup of banana, 3 dates.

7. Mixed berries, cashews & honey: ½ cup of mixed berries, 1 tsp. of cashews and 1 tsp. of honey.

8. Cacao powder, coconut oil & dates: 1 tbsp. of cacao powder, 1 tbsp. of coconut oil and 3 dates.

Jo's tips: Always add the eggs in towards the end of the blending and turn the speed down low. This way you will do the least amount of damage to the egg yolk.

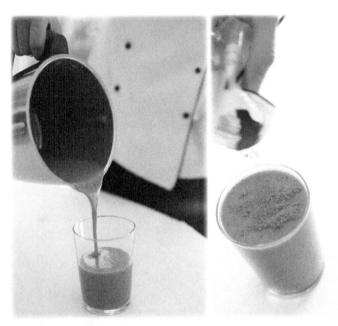

Method:

Place eggs, coconut water, coconut flesh, coconut oil and cinnamon in a blender and add selected fruit combination. Blend until smooth. For a chilled effect, blend a couple of ice cubes through it.

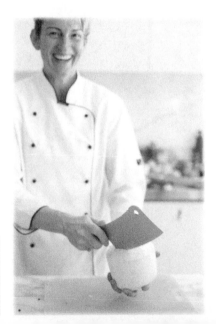

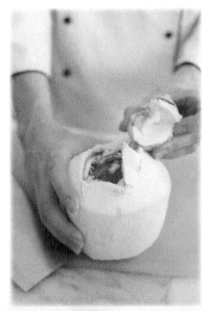

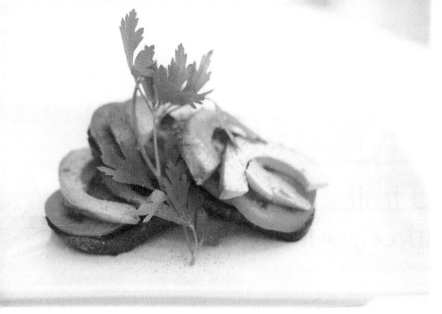

sliced tomato & avocado, cracked pepper on toasted sourdough

Serves one @ $2.75 per serve

½ - 1 sliced avocado
depending on the size
1 Truss or Roma tomato (sliced)
2 slices of fermented sourdough
(toasted)

Pinch of cracked pepper
Pinch of Celtic sea salt or Himalayan
rock salt
¼ fresh lemon wedge (optional)

Jo's tips: For all bread products: Make sure you source a good quality fermented sourdough, using the traditional fermentation methods. This will ensure the bread is nutrient-dense and easier on the digestive system. For those that are gluten intolerant, source a quality organic gluten free alternative such as buckwheat.

Method:

Layer the sliced tomato and avocado over the toasted sourdough. Squeeze over the lemon juice if desired and sprinkle with a pinch of salt and cracked pepper.

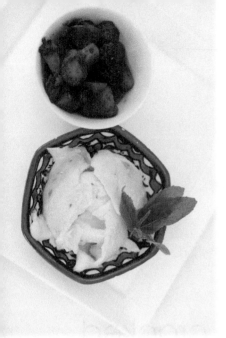

stewed fruit compote, cultured yoghurt & young coconut flesh

Serves one @ $2.90 per serve

1 cup of fresh
or frozen mixed berries
½ tsp. of cinnamon
2 tbsp. of cultured yoghurt

1 tbsp. of chopped
fresh coconut flesh
1 tsp. of shredded coconut
(toasted).

Jo's tips: The compote can be made ahead of time in bulk and stored in the fridge; however if you find yourself short of time, then use fresh mixed berries instead.

For cultured yoghurt, my preference is sheep's or goat's milk yoghurt or making your own with Cleopatra's raw milk. See instructions below:

Method:

Place the mixed berries and cinnamon into a saucepan and gently bring to a simmer. If using fresh fruit, add a tbsp. of water. When the fruit has come to a simmer, remove from heat and let cool.

Serve warm or chilled with yoghurt and coconut flesh separately, or on top sprinkled with toasted coconut.

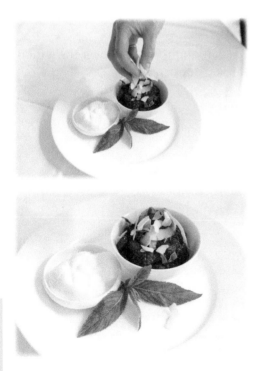

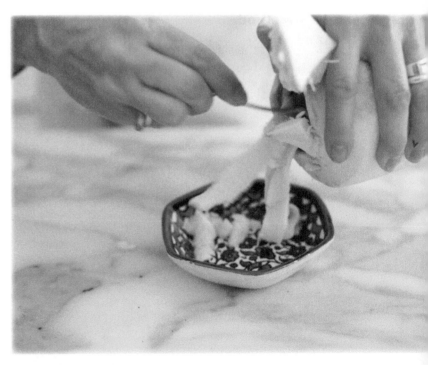

HOME MADE YOGHURT AND CHEESE

Makes approximately 10 serves @ $0.90 per serve

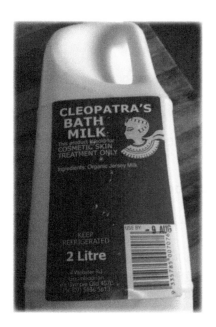

Ingredients:

- 2 litres of Cleopatra's raw bathing milk (sold for cosmetic purposes only and tastes delicious!)

Method:

Decant 2 litres of Cleopatra's Bath Milk into a glass jar and leave out on the bench until the whey separates from the milk solids (takes about 2 - 5 days depending on the temperature). Then line a colander with either muslin, or an old clean tea towel that has been wet and wrung out. Place colander over a glass bowl or stainless steel saucepan. Gently pour the milk solids and whey into colander, cover and allow straining for 2 days. The greenish colour liquid that has strained from the milk solids is your homemade whey - rich in good live bacteria. It will be preserved in the fridge for several months and can be used for making Beet kavas, and as a starter for fermented vegetables. Both recipes are included under Additional Recipes at the end of this 21-day meal plan.

Scrape the remaining milk solids (now resembling a firm yogurt / cheese curd) from the teatowel or muslin and transfer to a clean glass container and refrigerate. It will keep for about 2 weeks. Try adding some of your favourite fresh herbs and lemon juice to a serve of the cheese, and having it with sourdough or sprouted grain bread. You can turn the texture into a light yoghurt by mixing a little whey liquid through it, and adding a little honey or maple syrup, a pinch of cinnamon and vanilla powder.

QUARK CHEESE WITH SLICED TOMATOES ON TOASTED SOURDOUGH

Serves one @ $2.75 per serve

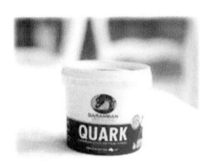

Ingredients:

- 2 tbsp. of quark cheese
- 1 Truss or Roma tomato (sliced)
- 2 slices of fermented sourdough (toasted)
- Pinch of cracked pepper
- Pinch of Celtic sea salt or Himalayan rock salt.

Jo's tips: Quark is a quality German style cheese that makes a far healthier and nutrient rich choice over commercial cottage cheese. Always choose the full fat option. Low fat and no fat products always have additional ingredients added back in such as sugar or other forms of carbohydrate to make up for the loss in taste and consistence when the fat component is removed.

Method:

Spread the quark cheese over the toasted sourdough, sprinkle a pinch of cracked pepper over the top, and then top with sliced tomato and a pinch of salt.

POACHED EGGS & BACON WITH STEAMED ASPARAGUS & CHERRY TOMATOES

Serves one @ $4.75 per serve

Ingredients:

- 2 eggs
- 2 rashers of bacon
- 3 asparagus stalks cut in half
- 2 cherry tomatoes sliced in half

Jo's Tip: Always try to source a nitrite free bacon product. There is no sense in adding to the toxins in your body. Your body works very hard to process and eliminate those toxins. This process requires energy, which most people are already lacking!

Method:

Using a double boiler or a stainless steel colander over a saucepan, bring 200ml of water to a boil, and steam the asparagus sticks at the same time as poaching the eggs.

Meanwhile place the bacon under a preheated grill and grill for approximately 3-5 minutes both sides depending on the thickness of the bacon.

Use either a poacher for the eggs or a sauté pan ¾ full with water and bring to boil. Add a tsp. of apple cider vinegar (this helps the eggs to stay together when you crack them into the water). Poach the eggs for 2 - 3 minutes, depending on how soft and running you like your eggs.

Serve and garnish with cherry tomatoes

APPLE & CINNAMON BUCKWHEAT PANCAKES WITH CULTURED YOGHURT & MAPLE SYRUP

Serves four @ $4.55 per serve

Ingredients:

- ¾ cup gluten-free all-purpose flour mix
- ¾ cup of buckwheat flour
- 3 tsp. of gluten-free baking powder
- 1 cup of coconut milk
- 2 eggs
- 2 tsp. of pure maple syrup
- Melted butter to grease.

Cinnamon apples:

- 2 apples (cored and thinly sliced)
- 1 tbsp. of cultured butter
- ½ cup of water
- 1.5 tbsp. of pure maple syrup
- ½ tsp. of ground cinnamon
- 8 tbsp. of cultured yoghurt.

Jo's Tips: This mixture can be made up to 24 hrs in advance and refrigerated. Make sure to whisk the mixture and rest it for a few minutes before use.

Rice or almond milk may be substituted for coconut and the apples may be substituted for sliced pear or the fruit compote.

Method:

Sift the combined flours and baking powder into a large bowl and make a well in the centre. (Alternatively, sift into a food processor).

In a separate bowl, whisk together the coconut milk, egg and maple syrup.

Gradually add the milk mixture to the flour mixture, whisking/blending constantly until smooth.

Set aside for 15 minutes to rest.

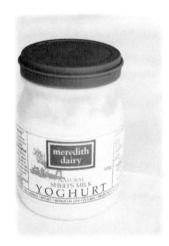

Meanwhile, to make the cinnamon apples, toss the thinly sliced apples in the cinnamon powder. Melt butter in a large saucepan and sauté the apples until just soft, add the maple syrup and water and bring to a simmer or until the liquid has reduced to syrup. Keep warm.

Brush a large non-stick frying pan with melted butter and heat over medium heat. Pour two 60ml (¼ cup) portions of batter into the pan, allowing room for spreading. Cook for 1 - 2 minutes, or until bubbles appear on the surface and pancakes are golden underneath. Turn and cook for a further 1 - 2 minutes or until golden. Transfer to a plate and cover with a clean tea towel to keep warm. Repeat, in 5 more batches, with the remaining batter to make 12 pancakes.

Divide pancakes among plates, top with apple mix and serve immediately with cultured yoghurt on the side.

"Australians have forgotten the art of turning leftovers into another meal and we throw out $8 billion of edible food each year."
- Sydney Morning Herald (23/12/12)

QUINOA PORRIDGE WITH NUTS, CULTURED YOGHURT AND A DRIZZLE OF HONEY

Serves one @ $3.30 per serve

Ingredients:

- ½ cup of organic quinoa (soaked over night)
- 1 ¼ cup of coconut milk
- 100 grams of fresh fruits (grated apple / pear / blueberry or strawberry)
- 20 grams of chopped organic almonds / walnuts / pecans (soaked over night)
- 1 tsp. of organic honey.

Jo's tips: Quinoa is a great alternative to rolled oats and a quick, easy and tasty way to get your protein in the morning if you're not such a savoury person at breakfast!

Method:

Rinse the now sprouted quinoa and transfer to a frying pan. Add coconut milk to cover the quinoa, bring to a simmer and cook the quinoa, the milk will be absorbed. Add a little extra water if the consistency is too thick

When quinoa has absorbed the milk, turn the heat to low and add the nuts and fruit.

Serve with a drizzle of honey and cinnamon.

SMOKED SALMON & AVOCADO, CRACKED PEPPER ON TOASTED SOURDOUGH

Serves one @ $3.80 per serve

Ingredients:

- 2 slices of smoked Salmon
- ½ avocado (sliced or mashed)
- 2 slices of fermented sourdough (toasted)
- Pinch of cracked pepper
- Squeeze of fresh lemon juice.

Jo's tips:Once again, sourcing a nitrate-free smoked salmon or using sashimi grade raw salmon instead of smoked salmon will prevent the intake of chemicals and toxins associated with smoked products.

Method:

Spread the avocado on the two slices of sourdough and lay the salmon on top. Sprinkle with pepper and a drizzle of lemon juice.

Do you know what you are really eating or where it comes from? Have you ever tracked your food back down the production line to see how, where, and from what your food is made?

HOMEMADE RAW COTTAGE CHEESE & HERBS, TOMATO, CRACKED PEPPER ON TOASTED RYE SOURDOUGH

Serves one @ $2.75 per serve

Ingredients:

- 2 slices of fermented Rye sourdough (toasted)
- 50g of homemade cottage cheese
- 1 tomato (sliced)
- Pinch of cracked pepper
- 1 tbsp. of fresh herbs
- Squeeze of fresh lemon juice.

Jo's tips: Parsley, coriander or thyme is a favourite of mine with this cheese. You can always substitute fresh herbs for dried herbs.

Method:

Mix the cheese with the lemon juice and herbs.

Spread the cheese evenly between the two slices of toasted sourdough. Place the sliced tomato evenly on top and sprinkle with black pepper

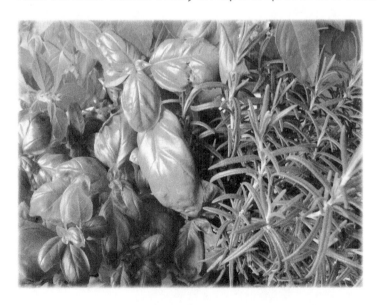

SOFT BOILED EGGS TOPPED WITH BUTTER & FRESH PARSLEY & STEAMED GREEN BEANS

Serves one @ $1.85 per serve

Ingredients:

- 2 eggs
- 1 tsp. of cultured butter
- 1 tsp. of chopped parsley
- 10 green beans, topped and tailed.

Jo's tips: I love this fast and simple breakfast that gives me the right combination of fuel to start my day. A quality source of protein, fat, and carbohydrate. I often use up leftover vegetables from the night before.

Method:

Place eggs in saucepan and cover with water, bring water to boil and boil eggs for 3 minutes. In the meantime, steam the green beans in a stainless steel colander over the eggs with a lid over the colander. Remove saucepan from heat, and set aside the green beans. Drain the boiling water and run the eggs under cold water for a few seconds. Using a knife, cut the top off the eggs and, with a teaspoon, gently empty the contents into a ramekin. Add the butter and parsley to the eggs and mix through.

Serve the green beans on the side.

SCRAMBLED EGGS AND CHIVES IN A THIMBLE OF SALMON GRAVLAX

Serves one @ $4.20 per serve

Ingredients:

- 2 eggs (whisked)
- 30g of ghee
- 50g of salmon gravlax
- 1 tbsp. of chives
- Pinch of Celtic salt and cracked pepper
- 2 slices of toasted sourdough.

Jo's tips: Definitely a weekend dish for when you have a little more creative time on your hands. The finished look is always so inviting and the flavours never disappoint!

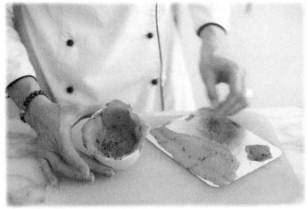
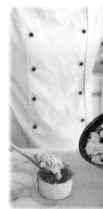

Method:

Line the ramekin with the salmon gravlax allowing the salmon to just sit over the edge of the ramekin, and set them aside.

Heat up a sauté pan on medium heat and melt the ghee. Add the chives to the butter. Add salt and pepper to eggs and pour into the pan of melted butter and chives. Scramble until soft. Fill the ramekin with the scrambled eggs mix and gently fold over the sides of the salmon to cover the eggs, as shown below. Turn the ramekin upside down on a serving plate and serve with toasted sourdough.

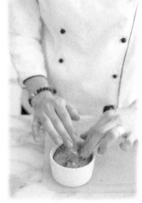
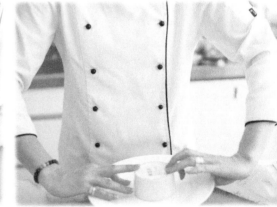

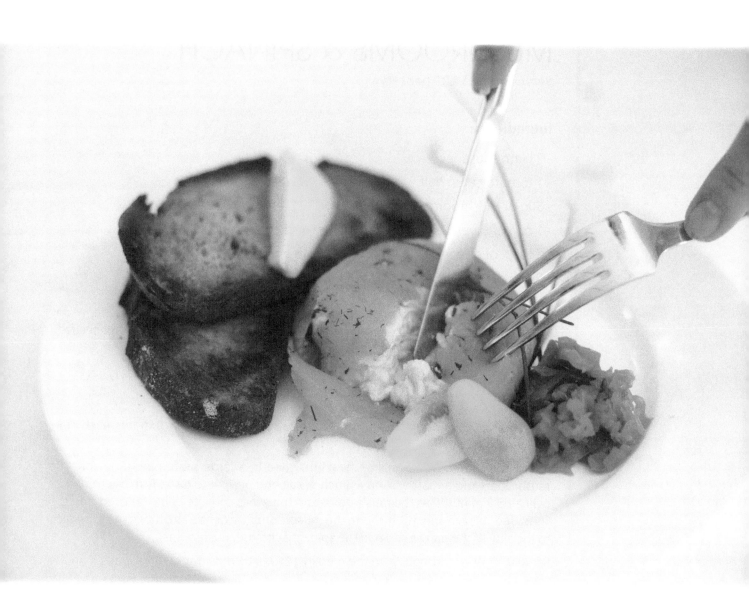

GRILLED LAMB SAUSAGES WITH A MEDLEY OF SAUTED TOMATOES, MUSHROOMS & SPINACH

Serves one @ $4.20 per serve

Ingredients:

- 2 lamb sausages
- 1 tomato cut in half
- 50g of mushrooms (sliced)
- 1 cup of silver beet spinach (washed and cut/shredded)
- 1 tbsp. of ghee
- Pinch of Celtic salt and cracked pepper.

Jo's tips: Be mindful to ask your butcher or organic meat supplier if the sausages have any gluten or natural preservative products. Many still do and, in my opinion, it is not needed. I have sourced excellent organic sausages without.

Method:

Grill the sausages under medium heat for approximately 5 - 8 minutes each side, depending on the thickness of the sausages.

Whilst the sausages are grilling, heat the ghee in a large sauté pan and sauté the mushrooms and tomatoes. Add a pinch of salt and pepper to taste. Turn the tomatoes over after 3 minutes. As the mushrooms and tomatoes come to being finished, add the shredded spinach and mix through the mushrooms (be gentle and move the tomatoes to the side of the pan as you mix the spinach with the mushrooms).

Serve the grilled sausages with the medley of tomato, mushrooms and spinach on the side.

ROASTED VEGETABLE AND BASIL FRITTATA

Serves four @ $ 2.15 per serve

Ingredients:

- 8 eggs whisked and seasoned with Celtic sea salt and cracked pepper
- 1tbsp. of ghee
- ½ onion (sliced)
- ½ cup of sweet potato, peeled, sliced and steamed (don't over-cook)
- ½ cup of broccoli florets steamed (don't over-cook)
- ½ cup of basil leaves roughly torn by hand.

Jo's tips: A frittata makes a great breakfast, lunch or dinner, and is a great way to use up leftover roast or steamed vegetable from another meal.

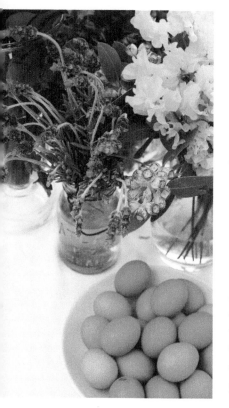

Method:

Pre-heat oven to 160 degree Celsius (160°C).

In a large sauté pan, melt the ghee and sauté the sliced onions for 2 minutes. Add the sliced potato and sauté for a minute on each side, then add broccoli and sprinkle over the basil. Pour over the egg mix and gently lift the contents of the pan so the egg mix can spread over the base of the pan. Allow the egg mix to slowly set, and then finish in either a pre-heated oven or under a grill. If using an oven, make sure the handle of the sauté pan is heat proof.

Serve hot or cold, with or without a mixed green salad.

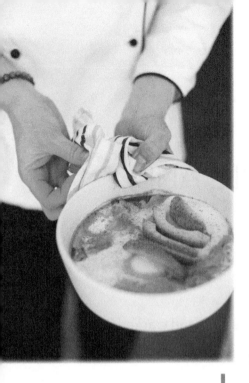

BAKED EGGS WITH TUSCAN HERBS & SHAVED LEG OF HAM

Serves one @ $3.95 per serve

Ingredients:

- 2 eggs

- ½ red onion (diced)

- 1 clove of garlic (chopped)

- ¼ avocado (sliced)

- 1 cup of pureed tomatoes

- 100g of shaved leg of ham

- 1 tbsp. of hand torn basil leaves

- 1 tsp. of Ovvio Tuscan herbs

- Celtic sea salt and cracked pepper to season

Jo's tips: One of the best Sunday brunch dishes EVER! I just love the flavours. I use my naturopath's organic Tuscan herbs (Ovvio), which are amazing.

Method:

Pre-heat oven to 220°C.

Butter a ceramic baking dish and line with shaved ham, onions, tomatoes, garlic, Tuscan herbs and a splash of water. Season well. Cover with baking paper and foil and bake for 15 minutes at 120°C. Remove from oven and remove cover. Create 2 small wells and crack an egg into each. Re-cover and continue baking until eggs are cooked with a soft yolk finish.

Serve with sliced avocado on top and fresh basil

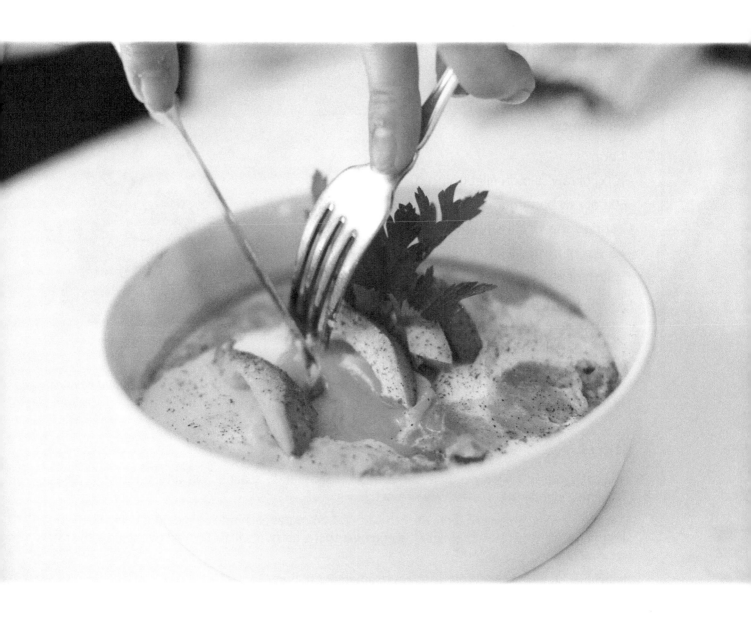

SALMON & DILL FISH CAKES SERVED WITH STEAMED KALE, TOPPED WITH FRIED EGG

Serves one @ $3.85 per serve

Ingredients:

- 1 egg
- 100g of raw salmon fillet (minced)
- 60g of raw barramundi fillet (minced)
- 2 spring shallots (finely chopped)
- 1.5 tsp. of fresh dill (chopped)
- Splash of filtered water
- 1 tbsp. of ghee
- 1 cup of kale (washed and chopped)
- Celtic sea salt and cracked pepper to season

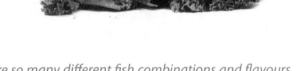

Jo's tips: Another Sunday brunch favourite! There are so many different fish combinations and flavours you could play with, even chopping prawns through the mix.

Method:

Using a splash of water, combine the salmon, barramundi, shallots, dill and seasoning. When completely blended, form the shape of a patty.

Heat ghee in a sauté pan and sauté the fish patty for 4 minutes each side on medium heat. When you turn the fish patty over, crack and fry the egg next to the patty. It will be cooked by the time the fish patty has finished cooking.

Meanwhile, steam the kale. This takes approximately 3 minutes.

To serve, toss the kale through some butter, and season with salt and pepper. Place the salmon patty on top. Then gently place the fried egg on top of the patty.

Serve immediately.

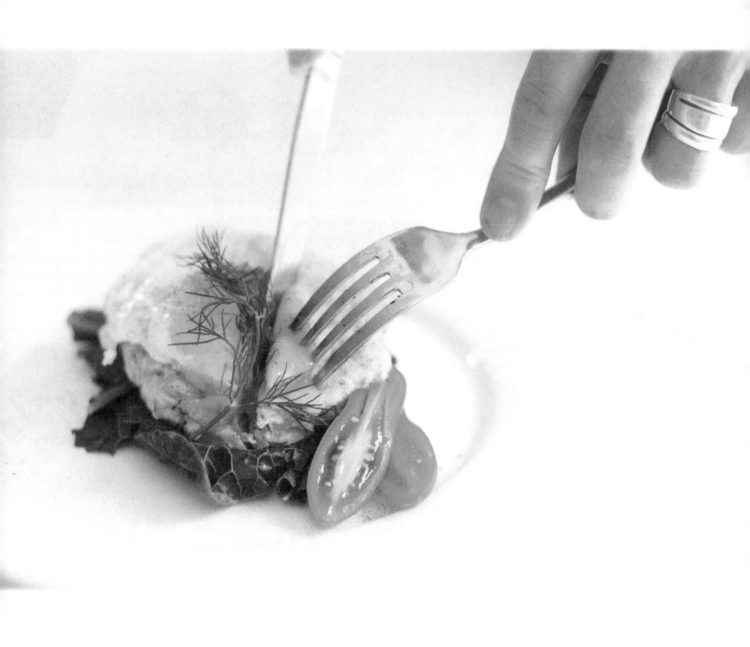

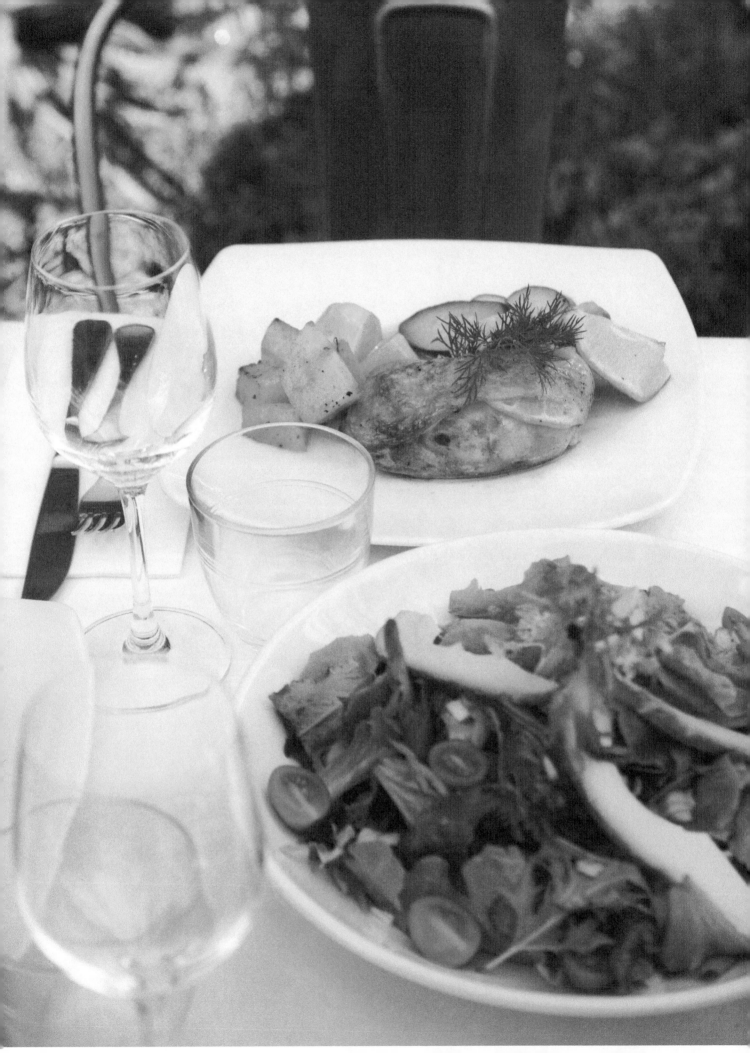

LUNCHES

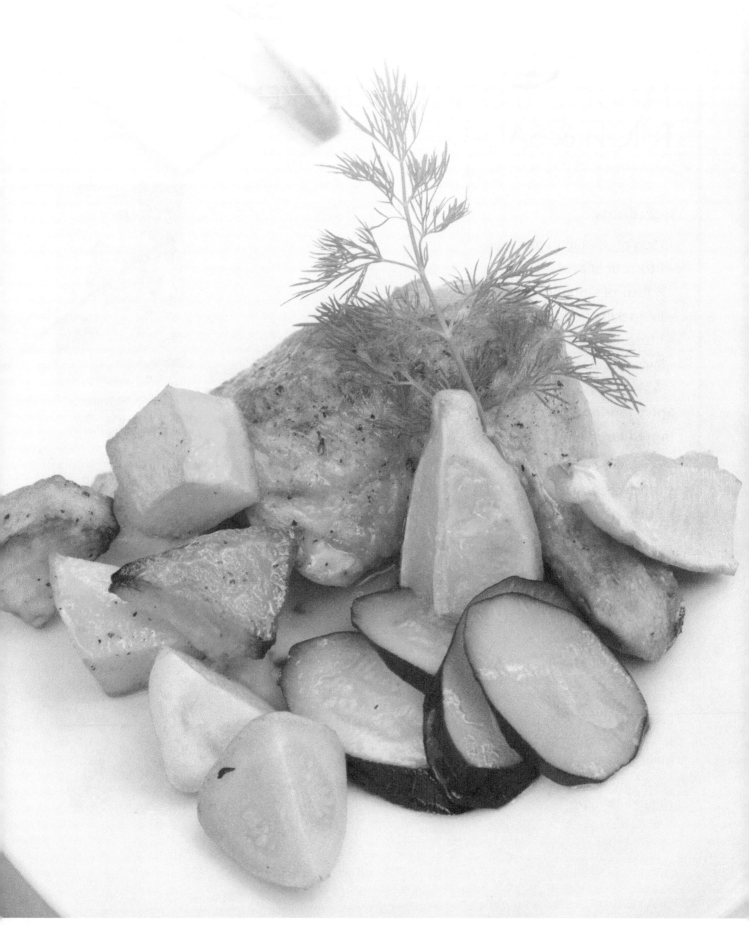

TANDOORI GRILLED CHICKEN THIGH & SALAD

Serves one @ $5.75 per serve

Ingredients:

- 150g of chicken thigh fillet
- 1 tbsp. of ghee
- ½ tbsp. of tandoori spice mix
- 1 ramekin of cultured yoghurt (optional)
- 1 tbsp. of fermented vegetable - see additional recipes
- Mixed salad - see additional recipes.

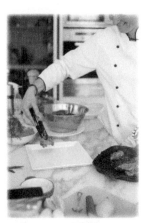

Spicy Tandoori Mix (Makes 3 ½ tbsp):

Ingredients:

- 2 tsp. of red chilli powder
- 1tbsp. of paprika
- 2 tbsp. of garam masala

Jo's Tips: If making your own tandoori mix seems too time consuming or overwhelming, pure food essentials and gourmet organic both do an organic tandoori spice mix.

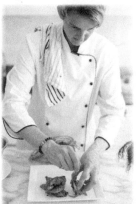

Method:

Combine chilli powder, paprika and garam masala. Use 1 recipe per 4 servings. Rub on to meat up to 1 day before, and on fish up to 2 hours before cooking. Spices will keep in sealed glass jar for up to 3 months.

In a stainless steel bowl, toss the chicken thigh in the tandoori spices.

Heat the ghee either on a cast iron grill plate or sauté pan. Cook the chicken thigh on medium heat for approximately 6 mins both sides.

Serve with mixed salad, a tbsp. of fermented vegetables and a small ramekin of cultured yoghurt.

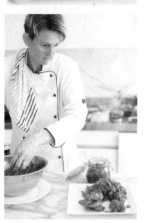

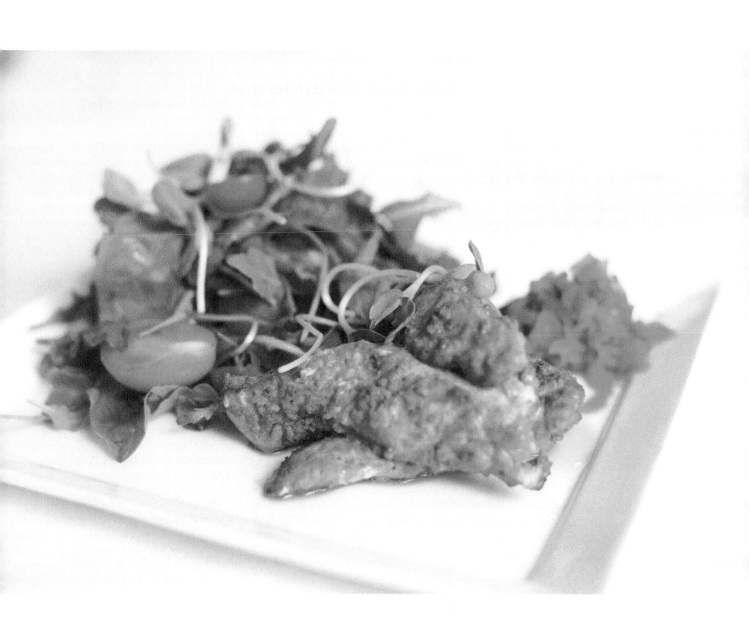

PRAWN AND AVOCADO SALAD

Serves four @ $5.25 per serve

Ingredients:

- 20 large ocean prawns, shelled and cleaned
- 1 mango (chopped)
- 1 avocado (chopped)
- 5 shallots (chopped)
- 6 cherry tomatoes (halved)
- ½ cup of fresh mint (chopped)
- 6 handfuls of baby spinach washed and ready
- 2 tbsp. of cold pressed olive oil
- Juice of 1 lemon
- 1 tsp. of raw honey
- 2 tbsp. of toasted coconut flakes.

Jo's tips: If mango is too sweet for you, then try a green pawpaw or even some pink grapefruit segments instead.

Method:

Make up the dressing by combining the olive oil, lemon juice and honey together in a sealed tight bottle and shake well.

In a large bowl, combine all other ingredients except toasted coconut flakes and pour the dressing over the top. Gently toss the salad so that the dressing is evenly spread.

Serve on a platter or individual plates and garnish with the toasted coconuts.

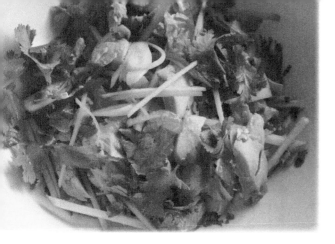

SALMON CUTLETS WITH GREEN APPLE SALAD

Serves four @ $8.25 per serve

Ingredients:

- 1 tsp Himalayan sea salt
- 4 salmon cutlets
- 2 medium apples sliced into match sticks
- 1 medium red onion (thinly sliced)
- 1½ cups of mint leaves
- ¾ cup of coriander leaves
- ½ cup of lime juice
- ¾ cup of raw cashew nuts.

Method:

Dressing: Combine the following in saucepan, bring to a simmer, remove and allow to cool before using.
- 1/3 cup rapudura sugar
- 2 tbsp. of tamari soy sauce
- 10g of fresh ginger.

Method:

Sprinkle salmon with sea salt.

Pan fry, grill or BBQ the salmon for approximately 4 minutes both sides.

Combine apple, onion, herbs, lime juice with ½ the dressing.

Either serve over cutlets or take the salmon off the bone and flake into the salad mix, sprinkle with nuts and drizzle the remainder of dressing on top.

GRILLED CHICKEN SAUSAGES WITH STEAMED VEGETABLES

Serves one @ $3.45 per serve

Ingredients:

- 2 chicken sausages
- 2 broccolini stalks
- ½ carrot (sliced into batons)
- 1 cup of sunflower sprouts washed and ready
- 1 tbsp. of fermented vegetables
- 1 tsp. of cultured butter

Jo's tips: Always ask your butcher if they add gluten or preservatives to their sausages. Even in organic sausages, gluten can be added through the flour they use to combine the mix.

Method:

Grill the sausages under medium heat for approximately 5 - 8 minutes each side, depending on the thickness of the sausages.

Whilst the sausages are grilling, simply steam the broccolini and carrots in a double boiler or in a stainless steel colander over boiling water with a lid.

Serve the chicken sausages with the vegetables and let the butter melt over the vegetables. Serve the fermented vegetable and sunflower sprouts on the side.

QUICK AND EASY TINNED TUNA OR SARDINES WITH A SUMMER SALAD

Serves one @ $3.55 per serve

Ingredients:

- 1 small tin of dolphin safe tuna.

Jo's tips: I don't make a habit of using tinned products and will only ever have a couple of tinned fish products on hand in case of an emergency!

When sourcing your preferred tinned fish, choose a fish that is responsibly caught; one that is non-farmed and environmentally friendly. Also make sure the fish isn't preserved in rancid vegetable oils like canola, cottonseed or soy bean. Natural brine or olive oil is the best option.

Method:

Serve with a summer salad. See additional recipes for summer salad.

To source food produced by farmers who respect and value nature is to enjoy food and know that it heals and nourishes more than just our bodies. It is food that is produced to restore and preserve our soils, oceans, and waterways and all that inhabits them.

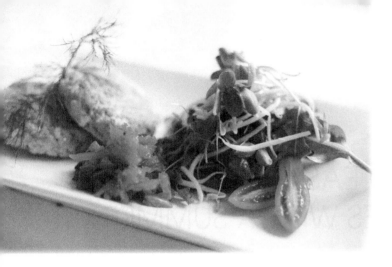

CHICKEN BURGERS AND SPRING SALAD

Serves five @ $5.75 per serve

Ingredients:

- 1 kg chicken mince
- 2 tbsp. of ghee
- 1 tbsp. of tomato paste
- 2 onions (finely chopped)
- 1 carrot (grated)
- 1 egg (beaten)
- 2 cloves of garlic (crushed)
- Celtic sea salt and pepper
- 1 handful of coriander (chopped).

Jo's tips: Lots of organic butchers offer cheaper prices per kg when buying in bulk, say about 2 kg. So try forms of mince that might have a special offer. Monetize wherever the opportunity presents itself!

Method:

Heat the ghee oil in a sauté pan.

Add onions and garlic; sauté for 2 - 3 minutes until soft. Remove from heat and combine with mince chicken and grated carrots.

Add tomato paste, salt and pepper, coriander and beaten egg.

Mix together until well combined.

Shape into burgers 5 x 200 grams burgers.

BBQ, grill or pan fry in a little ghee.

Serve with a spring salad and fermented vegetables. See additional recipes for spring salad and fermented vegetables.

GRILLED LEMON CHOUMOULA SQUID AND HERB SALAD

Serves four @ $3.25 per serve

Ingredients:

- 350g of squid tubes
- 1 lemon (peeled and chopped)
- 1 tbsp. of olive oil
- Celtic sea salt and cracked black pepper.

Jo's tips: Delicious when grilled on the BBQ.

Choumoula mix:

Makes 150ml of marinade for four servings of meat or fish.

Ingredients:

- 1 handful of flat-leaf parsley
- 1 handful of fresh coriander
- 4 garlic cloves (crushed)
- 1 tsp. of paprika
- 1 tsp. of cumin
- ½ tsp. of ground coriander
- ¼ tsp. of cayenne pepper
- 2 tbsp. of lemon juice
- 2 tbsp. of olive oil.

Method:

Open and score squid tubes. Cut scored tubes into 8 pieces. Toss in olive oil. Thread onto parallel skewers, with 2 pieces per pair of skewers. Grill on BBQ or ridged cast iron grill plate on top of the stove for 2 minutes on both sides.

Combine lemon with chamoula. Toss squid with chamoula and lemon to coat. Sprinkle with salt and pepper and serve hot with herb salad.

See Additional Recipes for herb salad.

STIRFRY CHICKEN, BROCCOLI, GINGER, SHALLOTS AND CASHEWS

Serves four @ $6.75 per serve

Ingredients:

- 600g of chicken thigh
- 2 tbsp. of coconut oil
- 1 bunch of spring onions (chopped)
- 1 head of broccoli cut into florets
- 1½ tbsp. of fresh ginger (grated)
- 1 red chilli (chopped) (optional)
- 2 cloves of garlic (crushed)
- 2 tbsp. of tamari soy sauce
- 1 bunch of coriander
- 2 tbsp. of honey (optional)
- 1 cup of raw cashew nuts.

Jo's tips: Replace the chicken for pork or beef. A variety of seasonal vegetables can be substituted in this dish, so be creative and use various combinations of your favourite vegetables. Also if needed, add a dash of chicken stock to the tamari for extra sauce

Method:

Heat the coconut oil over medium heat in a wok/fry pan.

Add onions, chilli and garlic, and ginger. Stir-fry for 2 - 3 minutes.

Add chicken and broccoli. Stir-fry for 2 - 5 minutes until chicken is cooked

If adding the honey, stir it into the tamari first.

Add the tamari, reduce for 1 minute.

Serve and garnish with fresh coriander leaves and raw cashews.

THAI BEEF SALAD

Serves four @ $6.70 per serve

Ingredients:

DRESSING:

- ¾ cup of lime juice
- 2 tbsp. of coconut sugar
- 4 tbsp. of fish sauce.

SALAD:

- 4 x 150g of eye fillet or sirloin steak
- 250g of bean shoots (washed and drained)
- 1/2 punnet of cherry tomatoes (halved)
- 1 small red onion, finely sliced
- 1 Lebanese cucumber sliced diagonally
- 1 cup of coriander, roughly chopped
- 1 cup of mint, finely chopped
- 4 kaffir lime leaves, sliced in fine strips
- 1 small red chilli, deseeded and finely chopped
- Raw unsalted peanuts (chopped) (optional).

Jo's tips: I prefer to make my own fish sauce, as commercially bought products tend to have MSG and lots of other preservatives, colourings and stabilisers. Not exactly Rocket Fuel!

I know traditionally palm sugar is used; however coconut sugar is packed with more minerals and therefore nutritionally holds more value.

Method:

Rub the beef with salt and pepper, add some coconut oil to a sauté pan and once the pan is hot, add the beef and seal on all sides. Cook until medium rare. Remove the meat and wrap in foil to retain the juices and leave aside to rest.

To make the dressing, dissolve the sugar in a bowl with the lime juice and fish sauce and set aside. In a large bowl add the bean shoots, tomatoes, onion, cucumber, coriander, mint, and chilli. Toss together.

Using a sharp knife, slice the beef as evenly and finely as you can and add to the salad mix. Pour the dressing over the salad, toss gently, and sprinkle with peanuts to garnish.

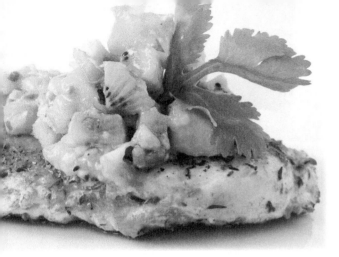

POACHED COCONUT CHICKEN WITH A TROPICAL SALSA

Serves four @ $7.25 per serve

Ingredients:

- 4 x 150g of chicken thigh
- 200ml of coconut milk
- Juice and zest of 1 lemon and 1 orange
- 2 star anise.

Salsa

- 2 mangos or ½ pineapple (cubed)
- Juice of 1 lemon
- 1 tablespoon of olive oil
- 1 avocado (cubed)
- 1 cup of bean sprouts
- 1 red onion (chopped)
- 1 red chilli (chopped)
- 1 handful of chopped coriander.

Method:

Marinate chicken in coconut, star anise and citrus up to 2 hrs.

Poach on medium heat for approximately 10 - 12 minutes in oven or covered in a sauté pan on the stovetop.

Reduce marinade to half and blitz in blender to get sauce smooth (optional).

For salsa, combine all ingredients and serve on the side or on top of chicken.

Serve with your choice of salad; I like the herb quinoa salad with this dish.

DINNER

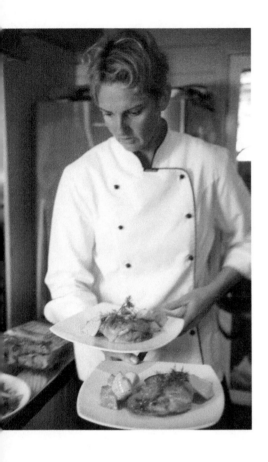

SLOW-ROASTED LEMON AND THYME CHICKEN

Serves four @ $6.75 per serve

Ingredients:

- 1 large whole chicken (this dish can also be done with individual cuts of chicken Maryland's -1 per person)
- 3 lemons (2 of them sliced and the 3rd cut in half if stuffing a whole chicken)
- 2 bunch of lemon thyme
- 2 cloves of garlic (sliced)
- Celtic sea salt and cracked pepper.

Jo's tips: As with most slow-cooked recipes, you can always seal the outside of the meat first before placing in slow cooker. However, if you are short of time, you can skip this step and it certainly won't detract from the taste. You may just be left with a faded colour to the skin of the chicken, that's all.

Method:

Carefully lift the skin away from the flesh and gently insert the sliced lemon, sprigs of thyme and garlic under the skin of the breast and legs. (Do likewise even if using chicken Maryland cuts).

Into the gut of a whole chicken, place the 2 halves of lemon each side and a whole bunch of thyme in-between. (Leave this step out if using chicken Maryland's).

Season with salt and pepper and place in slow cooker for up to 6 hrs on low heat for a whole chicken, and 4 hrs for chicken Maryland's. Alternatively cook slowly in a preheated oven on 120°C until tender.

Serve with roast mixed vegetables or salad.

LAMB MOUSSAKA WITH SALAD

Serves four @ $5.65 per serve

Ingredients:

- 1 large eggplant
- 500g of organic lamb mince
- ½ cup of melted ghee
- 1 tsp. of chopped garlic
- 1 large brown onion (diced)
- 1 cup of chicken broth
- 4 fresh tomatoes (diced)
- 3 tbsp. of tomato puree
- ¼ tsp. of pepper
- ½ tsp. of Rosemary
- ½ tsp. of basil
- 1 tsp. of parsley
- 8 ounces of quark cheese
- 1 egg
- 2 tbsp. of raw parmesan cheese
- Pinch of salt.

Jo's tips: This dish tastes even better the next day so make sure you make enough for leftovers!

Method:

Preparing your egg plant:

Slice the eggplant ¼ inch thick. Sprinkle evenly with salt. Transfer to a colander over a plate and set aside for 30 minutes to drain. This draws out the bitter juices.

Place the colander over a large bowl or in a sink. Carefully rinse each piece of eggplant under cold water, making sure you remove all the salt. Drain.

Transfer the rinsed eggplant pieces; a few at a time, to a clean work surface and pat dry with paper towel. Your eggplant is now ready to be used.

Brush both sides of eggplant with ghee, and bake on a sheet pan at 400 degrees, about seven minutes on each side. Eggplant should be sealed and partially cooked. Set aside.

For sauce, sauté onions and garlic in some ghee until soft. Add the minced lamb and cook for a further 3 - 5 minutes. Add chopped tomatoes, tomato puree, chicken broth, pepper, Rosemary, basil, parsley. Cook till thickened (about 20 mins).

Mix together the filling-quark cheese, egg, parmesan, and Rosemary.

Layer the ingredients in a glass or ceramic dish (start with ½ the mince sauce, then ½ eggplants, then ½ the cheese filling, and repeat).

Bake at 150°C for half an hour or so, until the filling is set.

Did you know that margarine decreases immune response?
"Pass the butter, please…"

AROMATIC COCONUT FISH CURRY

Serves four @ $7.85 per serve

Ingredients:

- 600g of skinless salmon fillets cut into cubes
- 2 tins of coconut milk
- 3 cups of snow peas or green beans topped and tailed
- 1 broccoli cut into florets
- 1 lemon grass finely chopped
- 1½ tbsp. of fresh ginger (grated)
- 1 red chilli (chopped) (optional)
- 1 clove of garlic (crushed)
- Juice of 1 large lime
1 bunch of coriander.

Jo's tips: Using salmon cutlets would make this dish even less expensive. You would just need to poach the cutlets whole.

The other fish that I love making this dish with are barramundi, snapper and cod.

You can also make the curry in a saucepan on the stovetop, simply follow the same process and allow the curry to simmer for ½ hr before adding the fish.

Method:

Place coconut milk, ginger, garlic, chilli, lemongrass and lime juice into a slow cooker and cook on low heat for 2½ hours.

Add salmon and vegetables, and continue cooking for 15 minutes.

Serve and garnish with fresh coriander leaves.

Herb quinoa makes a great compliment to this curry.

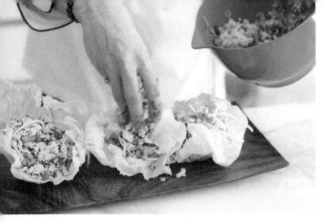

THAI CHICKEN LARB SALAD

Serves four @ $5.75 per serve

Ingredients:

- 600g of minced chicken
- 2 tbsp. of coconut oil
- 1 tbsp. of sesame seed oil
- Juice of 1 lime
- 1 bunch of spring onions (thinly chopped)
- 1 red chilli (chopped)
- 10g of ginger (thinly sliced)
- 2 cloves of garlic (chopped)
- Small knob of turmeric (thinly sliced) (optional)
- 1 large bag of bean sprouts
- 2 sticks of celery (thinly sliced)
- 1 Lebanese cucumber (finely diced)
- 1 handful of cherry tomatoes (halved)
- 1 red onion (finely diced)
- 1 handful of mint (chopped)
- 1 handful of coriander (chopped)
- 1 Iceberg lettuce - separate the layers into cups

Jo's tips: *This dish is fresh, tangy, full of fresh herbs and so easy to put together. Don't be put off by the amount of ingredients; you only have to sauté the mince, the rest is just 10 minutes of chopping and dicing!*

Method:

In a large sauté pan or wok, heat the coconut oil, and sauté the garlic, chilli, ginger, spring onions and turmeric for 2 minutes.

Add the chicken mince and work it until it has broken up and resembles a mince consistency.

In a separate bowl, combine all the other ingredients, adding the sesame seed oil and lime juice last, mix well for an even tangy taste. Mix chicken mince through the salad and serve by placing some of the salad mixture into the lettuce cups.

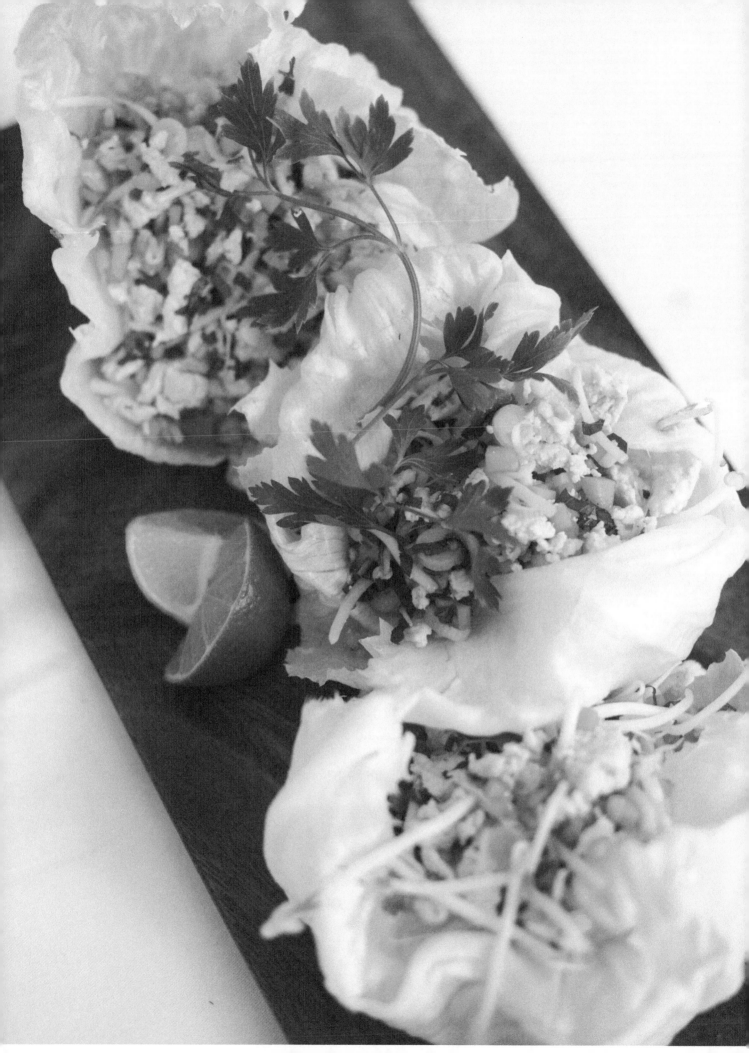

POACHED BARRAMUNDI INFUSED WITH GINGER, GARLIC & CORIANDER

Serves four @ $5.65 per serve

Ingredients:

- 4 x 150g of barramundi fillets
- 1½ tbsp. of fresh ginger (grated)
- 2 cloves of garlic (crushed)
- Juice of 2 limes
- ½ tbsp. of olive oil
- 2 handfuls of coriander.

Jo's tips: The quickest and easiest of One Pot wonders. It's awesome when cooking for one.

Method:

Use a double bowler or saucepan with a stainless steel colander. Line a double bowler with grease-proof paper (so that skin of fish doesn't stick to the base), ¼ fill with water and bring to boil.

Arrange fillets skin down over the paper. Make it so the fish is sitting in a little boat of greaseproof paper, so the juices don't run through.

Sprinkle over with ginger, garlic and lemongrass.

Pour in lime juice and olive oil, and pop the lid on and poach for 8 - 10 minutes till tender.

Garnish liberally with fresh herbs and serve with herb quinoa.

KANGAROO BURGERS WITH A PEAR & PERSIAN GOATS CHEESE SALAD

Serves five @ $3.00 per serve

Ingredients:

- 1kg of kangaroo mince
- 1 tbsp. of ghee
- 1 tbsp. of tomato paste
- 2 onions (finely chopped)
- 1 carrot (grated)
- 1 egg (beaten)
- 2 cloves of garlic (crushed)
- 1 tsp. of ground cumin
- Celtic sea salt and pepper
- 1 handful of mint (chopped).

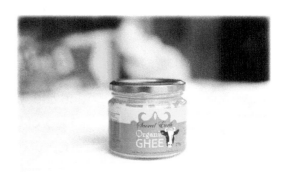

Jo's tips: Probably the cheapest wild non-organic meat you can buy!

Kangaroo is one of Australia's natural wild games, which we have in abundance. It is cleaner than commercially farmed cattle. This makes Kangaroo one of the more affordable natural game meats available to us all, even though it hasn't been certified as organic.

Method:

Heat the ghee oil in a sauté pan.

Add onions and garlic and cumin; sauté for 2 - 3 minutes until soft. Remove from heat and combine with kangaroo lamb and grated carrots.

Add tomato paste, salt and pepper, mint and beaten egg.

Mix together until well combined.

Shape into burgers 5 x 200g burgers.

BBQ, grill or pan fry in a little ghee.

Serve with a pear and Persian goat's cheese salad.

See additional recipes for pear and Persian goat's cheese salad.

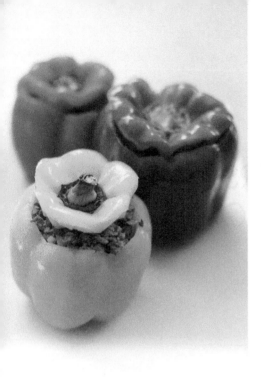

MEXICAN STYLE STUFFED PEPPERS

Serves four @ $4.75 per serve

Ingredients:

- 4 peppers (different colours)
- 2 tbsp. of olive oil
- 1 cup of chopped onions
- 6 tbsp. of chopped fresh parsley
- 2 garlic cloves (chopped)
- 1 tbsp. of sweet paprika
- 2 small red hot chillies (seeded and chopped)
- 1 tsp. of Celtic sea salt
- 1tsp. of ground black pepper
- 2 cups of chopped tomatoes
- 1 cup of stock (any kind is fine)
- 500g of minced beef.

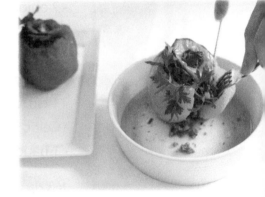

Jo's tips: You can also choose to make the filling with herb quinoa or a vegetable mix and then serve some protein on the side; however, I like the all in one approach!

Method:

Cut off the top (½ inch) of peppers and reserve. Scoop seeds from cavities. Brush the outside of the peppers with a little oil, then heat remaining oil in a large sauté pan over medium heat. Add onions, parsley, garlic, paprika, chilli, salt, and pepper. Sauté until onions have softened, then add meat and cook through until it is a crumbled mince consistency. Add the chopped tomatoes and stock. Simmer until the stock has almost reduced. The consistency should be moist but not running with liquid.

Fill pepper cavities with beef mixture. Stand filled peppers on a baking tray and put the tops back on. Bake on 150°C until peppers are tender (about 25 minutes).

Serve with your choice of salad.

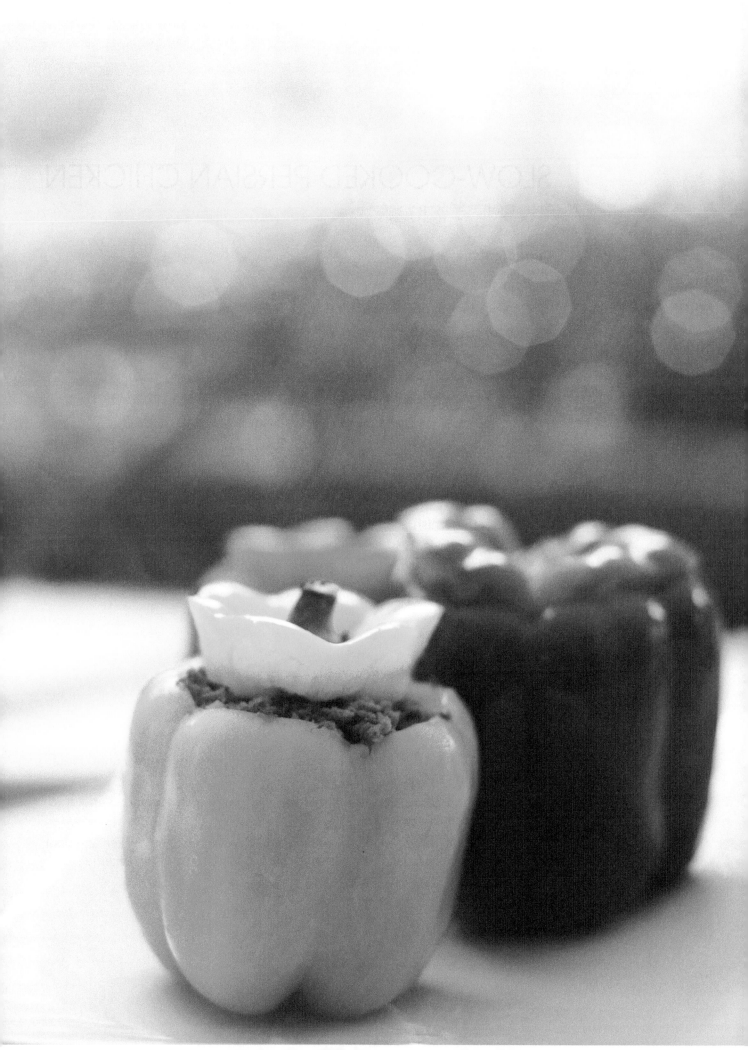

SLOW-COOKED PERSIAN CHICKEN

Serves four @ $4.95 per serve

Ingredients:

- 8 drumsticks
- 2 cups of quinoa (pre-soaked until sprouted)
- 2 tbsp. of coconut oil
- 2 tbsp. of Persian spice blend
- 1 large brown onion (diced)
- 2 cloves of garlic (crushed)
- 1200ml of chicken or vegetable stock
- 6 dates pitted and cut in half
- 50g of toasted almonds
- 4 tbsp. of parsley
- Coriander to garnish.

Jo's tips: Using chicken drumsticks makes this meal so affordable, not to mention just how much more nutrients you get when you choose cuts of meat that is on or close to the bone. Chicken Maryland or lamb chops is another great cut of meat for this dish.

Method:

Coat the chicken in the Persian spices and set aside.

In a large sauté pan, heat the coconut oil, add garlic, onions and cook until soft and lightly browned (about 6 - 8 minutes).

Add the chicken and seal and brown both sides.

Add 500ml of the stock and the dates and parsley, and bring to a simmer until chicken is tender (about 20 minutes).

Cook the quinoa separately in remaining stock for approximately 15 minutes until stock is absorbed and quinoa is tender.

Alternatively, if the sauté pan is large enough add the quinoa to the chicken and pour over enough stock to cover the chicken and quinoa, and finish cooking together.

Serve and garnish with toasted almonds and coriander.

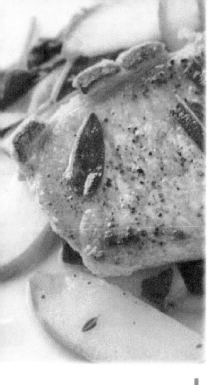

SLOW-COOKED SPICED PORK WITH APPLE AND FENNEL

Serves four @ $5.95 per serve

Ingredients:

- 4 large pork loin chops
- 2 apples (cored and sliced)
- 1 fennel (thinly sliced)
- 1 sprig of tarragon (stripped)
- 100ml of chicken stock
- **1½ tbsp. of Ovvio fragrant fruit herb & spice blend;** an aromatic dry blend of cinnamon, orange, clove, juniper & rosehip

Jo's tips: If you're local and can source Ovvio herbs (you can also purchase online), I grind this particular blend down into a finer consistency using a coffee grinder. Alternatively, create your own blend using the suggested fruits, herbs and spices.

Method:

Pour the stock into the base of a slow cooker. Coat the pork in the spices and arrange them in the stock. Arrange the apple, fennel and tarragon around the pork. Cover and set the slow cooker on low heat for 5 hrs.

Serve with your choice of freshly steamed seasonal vegetables with melted butter.

JO'S FISH PIE

Serves four @ $8.25 per serve

Ingredients:

- 2 tbsp. of ghee
- 1 brown onion (finely chopped)
- 100g of button mushrooms (quartered)
- 4 desire potatoes (thinly sliced)
- 12 green prawns
- 500g of skinned fish fillets cut into cubes (a mix of monkfish, salmon and cod)
- 2 tbsp. of fresh chervil (chopped)
- 1 tbsp. of fresh chives (chopped)
- 1 tbsp. of fresh parsley (chopped)
- Celtic sea salt and cracked black pepper to season
- 1 egg yolk (beaten with 1 tbsp. of water)
- 250ml of fish veloute.

To make veloute you need:

- 10g cultured butter
- 2 French shallots (finely chopped)
- 125ml of white wine
- 125ml of vermouth
- 250ml of fish stock
- 125ml of single cream
- 125ml of double cream
- Celtic sea salt and cracked black pepper to season.

Method:

Heat the butter in a sauté pan. Sauté onions till soft without colour (about 15 minutes).

Add wine and vermouth, and simmer till reduced by half (about 7 minutes).

Add stock, bring back to simmer and simmer again until reduced by half.

Stir in both creams, bring to a gentle simmer and reduce until the consistency is of a pouring cream. Season with salt and pepper.

Strain the sauce through a fine sieve. The veloute is now ready for use.

Jo's tips: If you're looking to impress friends for a dinner party, then this is the dish for it and it won't stretch your culinary skills too far either!

Other fishes suitable for this dish are snapper, barramundi and flat head.

Method:

Preheat oven to 160°C.

Heat ghee in a sauté pan and sauté onions until soft (about 5 minutes). Add mushrooms and cook for another 5 minutes. Set aside to cool.

In a rectangle glass pie dish, arrange the fish chunks on the base and scatter the herbs over the top. Season with salt and pepper and spoon over the onions and mushrooms, then add the fish veloute and gently mix together. Layer the sliced potato on top and gently brush with egg mix.

Bake in oven at 160°C temperature for 30 minutes, or until potatoes are golden brown.

Serve with freshly steamed broccolini and baby carrots.

BEEF CHEEKS WITH ONION, THYME & MUSHROOMS

Serves four @ $6.50 per serve

Ingredients:

- 1 tbsp. of coconut oil
- 800g of beef cheeks
- 12 French shallots (peeled but left whole)
- 200g of button mushrooms (halved)
- 1 leek (sliced)
- 2 large carrots (sliced)
- 3 bay leaves
- Sprig of thyme
- 2 star anise
- 1 garlic clove (sliced)
- ½ white pepper corns
- 350ml of veal or beef stock

Jo's tips: ATTENTION! This is REALLY IMPORTANT:

Please don't make the mistake of adding too much stock when using a slow cooker. The meat releases its own juice, which it cooks in. Adding too much stock will cause the meat to broil and turn out as tough as leather; not the purpose of slow cooking!

Method:

Seal and brown meat first (optional), then place meat in slow cooker.

Sauté onions, leek and mushrooms in coconut oil until lightly browned.

Arrange the onions and mushrooms on top along with the rest of the ingredients.

Pour in the stock.

Turn on to low heat and cook for 4 - 6 hours.

Serve with fresh, steamed seasonal vegetables.

CHICKEN & VEGETABLE CURRY

Serves four @ $6.75 per serve

Ingredients:

- 1kg of skinless chicken thigh fillets (cut in 1 inch strips or chunks)
- 1 large sweet potato (chopped into cubes)
- 2 large onions (quartered and sliced thinly)
- 3 cloves of garlic (minced)
- 1 tbsp. of Tamari soya sauce
- 2 tsp. of Madras curry powder
- 2 tsp. of chilli powder
- 1 tsp. of fresh turmeric (chopped)
- 1 tsp. of ground ginger
- 1 tsp. of Celtic sea salt
- ½ cup of chicken stock
- ½ cup of coconut cream.

Jo's tips: Again, using 2 drumsticks per person would reduce the cost of this meal. However, it wouldn't provide as much protein per person. I prefer chicken thigh to any other meat for this dish.

Method:

Mix all ingredients together in a slow cooker or Crockpot. Cover and cook on low heat for 3 - 4 hours or until chicken is tender.

Serve with your choice of fresh seasonal vegetables.

POACHED SNAPPER WITH LEEK AND FENNEL

Serves four @ $6.95 per serve

Ingredients:

- 4 x 150g of snapper fillets
- 1 fennel bulb (finely sliced)
- 1 leek (finely sliced)
- 1 garlic clove (finely chopped)
- 1 tsp. of grated turmeric root
- 1 tsp. of ginger (finely sliced)
- 100ml of fish stock
- 1 tbsp. of cultured butter
- Handful of fresh chives and coriander.

Jo's tips: Another great One Pot wonder, and you can easily substitute the fish with another white fleshing fish of your choice without detracting from the flavours created by the leek and fennel combination.

Method:

Using a saucepan with a stainless steel colander or double bowler, line the base or colander with grease-proof paper so that skin of fish doesn't stick to the base. Bring water to the boil.

Arrange fillet skins down over the paper. Make it so the fish is sitting in a little boat of greaseproof paper, so the juices don't run through.

Sprinkle the fennel, leek, garlic, ginger, turmeric and butter over the fish.

Pour in fish stock, then put the lid on and poach for 8 - 12 minutes till tender.

Garnish liberally with fresh herbs.

Serve fresh with your choice of fresh seasonal vegetables.

BRAISED DUCK WITH FIGS, HONEY AND VINEGAR

Serves four @ $8.15 per serve

Ingredients:

- 1 whole duck cut into portions (simple ask your butcher to do this for you)
- 2 tbsp. of ghee
- 2 red onions (chopped)
- 8 fresh figs (halved)
- 2 tsp. of lemon thyme (chopped)
- 2 sprigs of Rosemary
- 1 lemon peel cut into strips
- 1 orange peel cut into strips
- ½ stick of cinnamon
- 1¼ cup of chicken stock
- 2 tbsp. of raw honey
- 2 tbsp. of aged red wine vinegar.

Jo's tips: One of the more expensive of meals but the price of duck will vary anything up to $10 in price for a whole bird, depending on your provider. So shop around; it's worth it.

Method:

Heat 1 tbsp. of ghee in large sauté pan and sauté the onions.

When onions are soft and translucent, add the figs and seal.

Transfer the onions and figs into your slow cooker or Crockpot.

Add the remaining tbsp. of ghee to the pan and seal the duck pieces on all sides.

Arrange the duck on top, bringing some of the pieces of fig to the top.

Add the lemon and orange peels, thyme, and 1 sprig of Rosemary.

Add the vinegar and cinnamon quill.

Pour in the stock and strip the second sprig of Rosemary and sprinkle it over the top.

Drip the honey all over the duck.

Set your slow cooker on low heat and cook for 3 - 4 hours. Or cook slowly in crockpot in preheated oven 120 C for until tender

Serve with your choice of fresh, steamed seasonal vegetables.

POACHED LEMON MYRTLE CHICKEN WITH BRAISED VEGETABLES

Serves four @ $6.85 per serve

Ingredients:

- 4 chicken breasts
- 1300ml of chicken stock
- 1 carrot peeled and cut into quarters
- 1 parsnip peeled and cut into quarters
- 2 shallots
- 4 wedges of pumpkin (approximately 50g each)
- Wedges of sweet potato (approximately 50g each)
- 4 leaves of kale or silver beet
- 4 sprigs of lemon thyme (stripped)
- 4 lemon myrtle leaves (chopped)
- 4 sprigs of parsley (chopped)
- 2 bay leaves
- Celtic salt and pepper.

Jo's tips: I just love this dish! It's light, yet warming and fulfilling on a winter's day. You could easily substitute the chicken for a white fish like cod or barramundi and still keep everything else the same.

Method:

Arrange all veg except kale in a deep tray. Season with salt and pepper. Sprinkle with some thyme and 1 chopped lemon myrtle leaf on top.

Add 300ml of stock and braise in 150 C for 20 minutes until coloured and tender.

Add the kale or silver beet in the last 2 minutes to wilt it a little.

Rub the chicken breast with salt, pepper, thyme, and parsley and lemon myrtle.

Seal in a medium hot pan until it is golden brown, then place in a deep tray.

Pour remaining stock into pan and poach chicken in oven for 10 minutes whilst vegetables are braising.

To serve, place vegetables in a deep soup plate and top with chicken that has been sliced at an angle and fanned over the top of the vegetables. Pour some of the poaching stock over the top and garnish with sprig of thyme or parsley.

SLOW-ROASTED ROLLED LEG OF LAMB WITH ROSEMARY AND GARLIC

Serves about four to five @ $6.95 per serve

Ingredients:

- 1.5kg rolled leg of lamb
- 1 large sweet potato (chopped)
- 1 leek chopped into thick slices
- 1 large beetroot chopped into quarter wedges
- 2 cloves of garlic peeled and sliced in half
- 3 sprigs of Rosemary cut into smaller sprigs
- Celtic sea salt and black pepper to season.

Jo's tips: This just doesn't get easier. Follow the link to YouTube and watch how quickly I put this dish together! Great for feeding the family mid week or as a weekend roast.

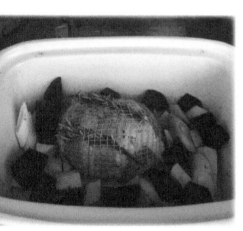

Method:

 Watch it on YouTube ←

Make small incursions into the flesh of the rolled leg of lamb and insert a piece of sliced garlic and a sprig of Rosemary. Repeat this evenly over the surface of the lamb.

Place the lamb in a slow cooker along with the chopped vegetables. Put the lid on and slow cook for 5 - 6 hrs on low heat.

Serve with some fresh, steamed seasonal greens.

'Please scan this QR code with your iphone to watch the you tube demonstration of this dish'

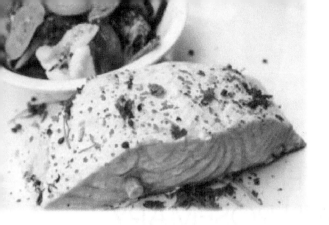

POACHED SALMON INFUSED WITH FRESH GINGER, LEMONGRASS AND MINT

Serves four @ $5.65 per serve

Ingredients:

- 4 x 150g of salmon cutlets
- 1½ tbsp. of fresh ginger (grated)
- 1 tender end of a lemongrass stalk (finely chopped)
- Juice of 1 lemon
- 1 tbsp. of olive oil
- 1 handful of mint (chopped).

Jo's tips: Another light, fresh dish that you could substitute with nearly any fish that is your favourite and still enjoy the flavours created in this dish.

Method:

Using a saucepan with a stainless steel colander or double bowler, line the base or colander with grease-proof paper so that skin of fish doesn't stick to the base. Bring water to the boil.

Arrange fillet skins down over the paper. Make it so the fish is sitting in a little boat of greaseproof paper, so the juices don't run through.

Sprinkle the ginger and lemongrass on them.

Pour it the lemon juice and olive oil, put the lid back on and poach for 8 - 12 minutes till tender.

Garnish liberally with fresh mint.

Serve with herb quinoa.

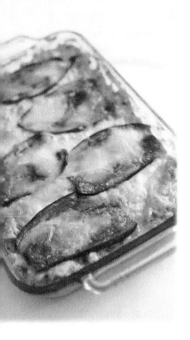

CHICKEN MOUSSAKA & SALAD

Serves four @ $6.85 per serve

Ingredients:

- 500g organic chicken mince
- ½ cup of melted ghee
- 1 tsp. of chopped garlic
- 1 large brown onion (diced)
- 1 cup of chicken broth
- 4 fresh tomatoes (diced)
- 3 tbsp. of tomato puree
- ¼ tsp. of pepper
- 1 tsp. of thyme
- 1 tsp. of basil
- 1 tsp. of parsley
- 8 ounces of quark cheese
- 1 egg
- 2 tbsp. of raw parmesan cheese
- Pinch of salt.

Jo tips: Very similar to the lamb moussaka and, again, even more flavoursome the next day. Be creative with your choice of herbs and don't let any recipe limit your innate intuition for other suitable ingredients. Recipes are a guideline and framework. Learn to bring your own personality to what you're creating!

Method:

Preparing your egg plant:

Slice the eggplant ¼ inch thick. Sprinkle evenly with salt. Transfer to a colander over a plate and set aside for 30 minutes to drain. This draws out the bitter juices.

Place the colander over a large bowl or in a sink. Carefully rinse each piece of eggplant under cold water, making sure you remove all the salt. Drain.

Transfer the rinsed eggplant pieces; a few at a time, to a clean work surface and pat dry with paper towel. Your eggplant is now ready to be used.

Brush both sides of eggplant with ghee, and bake on a sheet pan at 400 degrees, about seven minutes on each side. Eggplant should be sealed and partially cooked. Set aside.

For sauce, sauté the onions and garlic in some ghee until soft. Add the minced chicken and cook for a further 3 - 5 minutes. Add chopped tomatoes, tomato puree, chicken broth, pepper, thyme, basil and parsley. Cook till thickened (about 20 mins).

Mix together the filling, quark cheese, egg and parmesan.

Layer the ingredients in a glass or ceramic dish (start with ½ the mince sauce, then ½ eggplants, then ½ the cheese filling, and repeat).

Bake at 120°C for ½ hour or so, until the filling is set.

Serve with some fermented vegetables and mixed salad leaves.

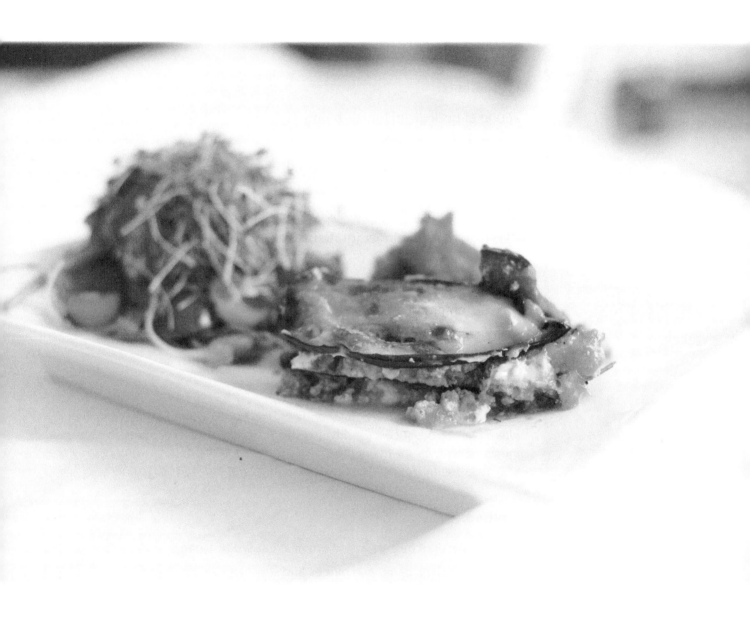

STIRFRY PORK WITH FRESH GINGER CHILLI AND GARLIC

Serves four @ $6.95 per serve

Ingredients:

- 600g of pork diced for stir-frying
- 1 large tbsp. of coconut oil
- 1 bunch of spring onions (chopped)
- 1 red pepper with seeds removed (chopped)
- 1 head of broccoli cut into florets
- 1½ tbsp of fresh ginger (grated)
- 2 red chilli (chopped)
- 2 cloves of garlic (crushed)
- 2 tbsp. of tamari soy sauce
- ¼ of chicken stock
- 1 bunch of coriander
- 1tbsp. of honey (optional)

Jo's tips: Who doesn't like a quick and easy stir-fry? Try using sesame seed oil as an alternative to coconut oil; the flavour is stronger and tastier. Keep your temperature moderate with all stir-frying otherwise you damage the nutrients and destroy the enzymes essential for digesting and absorbing what the food has to offer.

Method:

Heat the coconut oil over a medium heat in a wok/fry pan.

Add onions, chilli, garlic, and ginger, and stir-fry for 2 - 3 minutes.

Add range pork and broccoli; stir-fry for 2 - 5 minutes.

Add the stock and reduce for 1 minute, then add the tamari, stirring to mix with the stirfry.

If adding the honey, stir it into the tamari soy sauce first.

Serve and garnish with fresh coriander leaves.

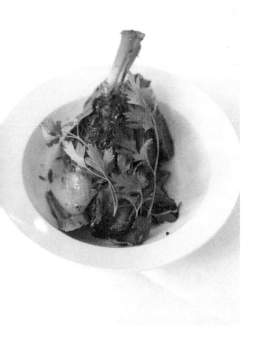

SLOW-COOKED LAMB KASHMIR SHANKS

Serves four @ $7.20 per serve

Ingredients:

- 4 lamb shanks
- 100ml of chicken stock
- 2 large carrots sliced approximately an inch thick on an angle
- 2 brown onions peeled and quartered

For the marinade:

- 1 large knob of ginger
- 3 cloves of garlic
- Juice of 2 lemons
- 1 tsp. of sea salt
- 1 tbsp. each of cumin and turmeric (ground)
- 1 tsp. each of cinnamon, black pepper, cardamom seeds (no husks)
- 3 dried chillies (crushed)
- ¼ cup each of soaked cashews and pistachio (crushed)

Jo's tips: You can always buy a pre-blended spice mix if making your own seems too tiring. You could simplify this dish by substituting the marinade ingredients with some fresh thyme and Rosemary and garlic.

Method:

Blend all ingredients together to form paste and rub over shanks.

Marinate for 2 hours.

Place in slow cooker with a little chicken stock, sliced carrot and quartered onions. Cook for 5 - 6 hours on low heat.

Garnish with fresh parsley and serve with a green salad.

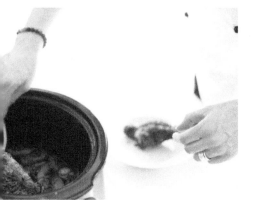

SNACKS

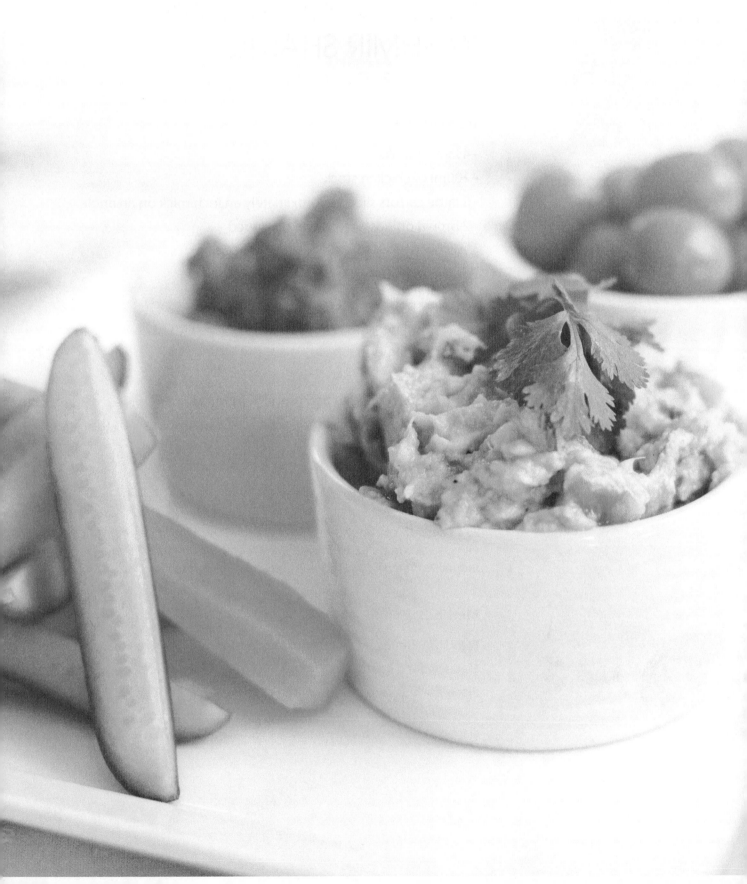

CHICKEN LIVER PATE

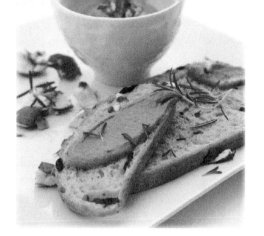

Serves six @ $2.15 per serve

I love sharing this recipe as it never ceases to amaze me how many people consider Chicken Liver Pate to be unhealthy. It was once considered the number one brain food and was always highly recommended for mums-to-be. Where did all this wisdom go? Now we consider it to be a sinful indulgence that clogs the arteries - what nonsense! On the contrary, with well sourced quality ingredients, it's jam-packed full of essential nutrients and is on my list of Super Foods for the following reasons:

It's rich in:

1. Iron for healthy blood.

2. Folate for healthy cell regeneration and protection from heart disease.

3. Vitamin B12 for a healthy nervous system.

4. Vitamin B6 for healthy hormones and protein metabolism.

5. Vitamin A for healthy eyes, skin and respiratory tract.

6. Zinc for healthy skin and immune system.

7. Protein for growth, repair and regeneration.

8. Choline (amino acid) for healthy nerves and muscles.

9. Cholesterol (yes, cholesterol IS an essential 'nutrient'. Without it, there'd be no steroid hormones, no estrogen, progesterone or testosterone. You'd have leaky cells and you wouldn't be able to store memories or make myelin which protects your nerves. If your cholesterol level is high, you need to find out why YOUR liver is producing more than it should. Your liver makes 80% of the cholesterol found in your body, 10% is made in your digestive tract and 5% in your skin. Only 5 - 10% comes from dietary sources).

The fat of breast milk contains more cholesterol than any other food! Did Mother Nature get it wrong? I think not.

Ingredients:

- 500g of organic chicken livers (it is most important to use organic liver only. It is the detoxifying organ after all)
- 1 onion (diced)
- 3 slices of bacon (optional)
- 1 clove of garlic
- 250g of organic butter
- 100ml of white wine (optional)
- Herbs such as rosemary, thyme, tarragon, or parsley (chopped) (optional)

Jo's tips: Don't overcook the livers; seal them both sides and then remove from heat. Blend all ingredients when cooled.

Method:

Heat 60g of butter in pan; add onion and garlic and sauté for 1 minute. Add bacon and chicken livers and sauté till opaque, then remove from pan and set aside to cool. Meanwhile, add herbs if selected and white wine to the onions and garlic and reduce to just a moist consistency. Let cool.

Transfer all ingredients to blender, add remaining butter and blend till smooth.

Transfer to glass container and refrigerate.

Additional melted butter can be drizzled over the top to preserve colour and help to keep the pate from forming a skin on top.

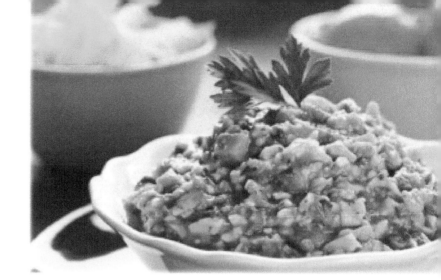

GUACAMOLE

Serves four @ $ 1.10 per serve

Ingredients:

- 2 avocados (mashed)

- ½ Spanish onion (diced)

- 2 tomatoes (chopped)

- 1 handful of chopped coriander leaves

- Roots from the coriander

- Juice of 1 lime

- 1 large clove of garlic (minced)

- 1 green chilli (chopped) (keep seeds if you like it hot)

- Celtic sea salt and pepper to season.

Jo's tips: Using a pestle and mortar to grind the coriander roots with the chilli, garlic, and lime juice is definitely what makes this yummy snack come alive. Blending in a food processor just doesn't give the same result.

Method:

Mix the lime juice, garlic, green chilli and roots of the coriander in a mortar and pound with a pestle until it is a fine paste. Mix the paste through the mashed avocado and then add the onion, tomatoes, salt and pepper and coriander leaves to the avocado. Mix together.

Serve with vegetable sticks or corn chips.

It can be stored in sealed glass container in the fridge for up to 3 days.

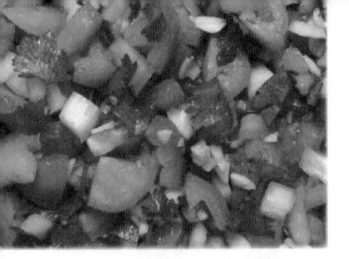

SALSA

Serves four @ $1.10 per serve

Ingredients:

- 4 truss or Roma tomatoes (chopped)
- 1 cup of basil (chopped)
- ½ Spanish onion (finely diced)
- 1 garlic clove (finely chopped)
- 100ml of olive oil
- Juice of ½ lemon
- 1 red chilli (de-seeded and finely chopped)
- Celtic sea salt to season.

Method:

Using a stainless steel or glass bowl, simply combine all ingredients together. Serve with corn chips or vegetable sticks.

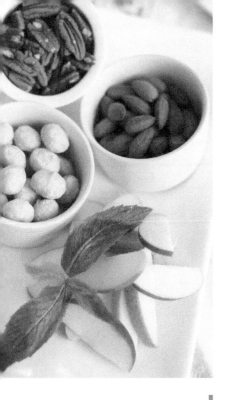

CRISPY ACTIVATED ALMONDS

Makes 33 portions @ $0.50 per portion

Ingredients:

- 1kg pack of almonds
- Filtered water
- 1 tbsp. of Celtic sea salt.

Jo's tips: No need to wash the salt off after soaking since this gives the nuts a great salty crunch when they are done. Follow the same method for all nuts. The only thing that will change will be the length of time it takes them to dry out. Macadamia nuts being the longest, at about 3 days.

Method:

Soak the almonds in a stainless steel or glass bowl for up to 24 hour or at the least overnight. Drain the nuts off the water in a colander. Dry the nuts out in a dehydrator by spreading the nuts evenly amongst the layers of the dehydrator with the temperature at 50°C and no hotter. The nuts are done when they are crunchy to the bite. This should take approximately from 24 - 48 hours.

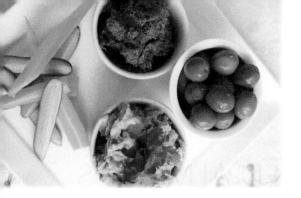

BABA GHANOUJ (EGGPLANT DIP)

Serves four @ $1.55 per serve

Ingredient:

- 1 or 2 eggplants (total of 1kg)
- 3 tbsp. of Extra Virgin olive oil
- 2 - 3 tbsp. of roasted tahini (sesame paste)
- 1 - 2 garlic cloves (more or less, depending on how garlicky you want your baba ghanouj to be) (finely chopped)
- 1 tsp. of ground cumin
- Juice of one lemon (about 2½ tbsp.)
- Salt and cayenne pepper to taste
- 1 tbsp. of chopped parsley.

Method:

Pre-heat oven to 180°C. Poke the eggplants in several places with a fork. Cut the eggplants in half lengthwise, and brush the cut sides lightly with olive oil (about 1 tbsp.) Place on a baking sheet, cut side down, and roast until very tender (about 35 - 40 minutes). Remove from oven and allow to cool for 15 minutes.

Scoop the eggplant flesh into a large bowl and mash well with a fork. Combine the eggplant, minced garlic, remaining olive oil (about 2 tbsp.), tahini, cumin, and 2 tbsp. of the lemon juice, the salt, and a pinch of cayenne. Mash well. You want the mixture to be somewhat smooth but still retaining some of the eggplant's texture.

Allow the baba ghanouj to cool to room temperature, then season to taste with additional lemon juice, salt, and cayenne. If you want, swirl a little olive oil on the top. Sprinkle with fresh chopped parsley.

Can be stored in a sealed glass container in the fridge for up to 5 days.

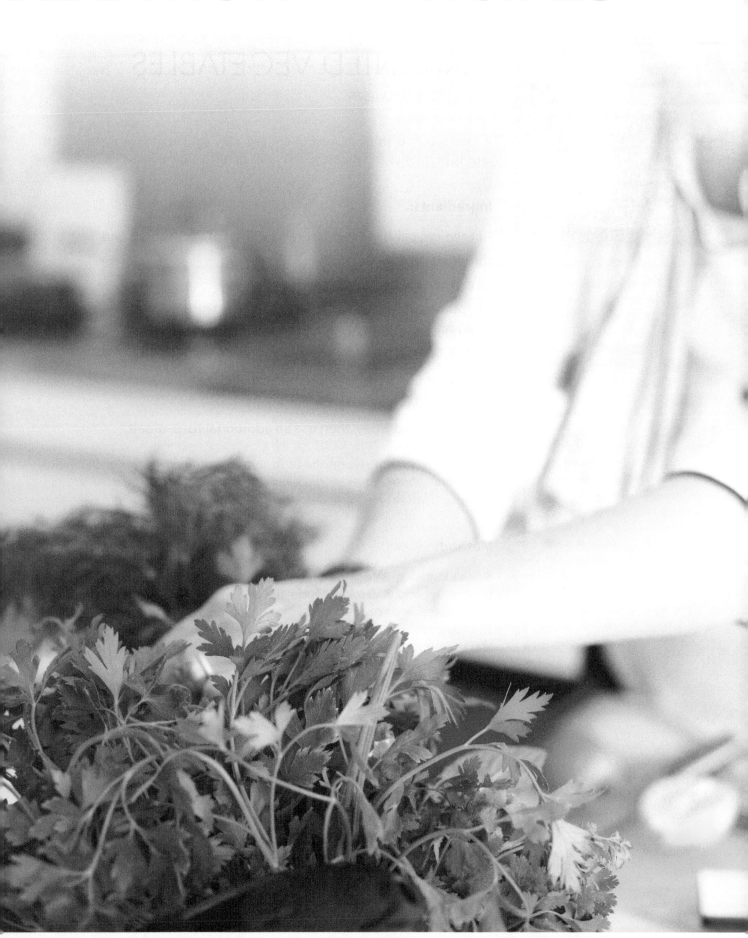

ADDITIONAL RECIPES

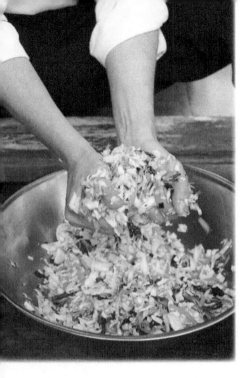

FERMENTED VEGETABLES

Fills a 2-litre Mason jar.

A tablespoon with each main meal provides your digestive system with quality probiotics and digestive enzymes that aid digestion.

Ingredients:

- 1 medium cabbage (red or green, or half of each) cored and shredded
- 3 carrots (grated)
- 1 apple (grated)
- 1 fennel (shredded) (optional)
- 2 tbsp. of caraway seeds
- 1 tbsp. of Celtic sea salt or Himalayan rock salt
- 4 tbsp. of whey as a starter (optional)
- If you have no whey, then use an additional tbsp. of salt.

Jo's tips: Be sure to release the build up of pressure in the jar in the initial fermenting phase, either in morning or evening. The fermentation process creates gas inside the jar that needs to be released.

Method:

Mix all ingredients together in a large bowl. Pound with a pestle or meat hammer for about 10 minutes until the juices start to release. Place in a large 2 litre mason jar and press down firmly until juices come to the top of the mix. The mixture should be, at least, 1 inch below the juices. Cover the jar tightly and keep at room temperature for 3 - 5 days before transferring to the fridge. Be sure to release the build up of pressure in the jar in the initial fermenting phase, either in the evening or in the morning.

Fermented vegetables will last for up to 3 months in the fridge.

→ **Watch it on YouTube** ←

'Please scan this QR code with your iphone to watch the youtube demonstration of preparing Fermented Vegetables

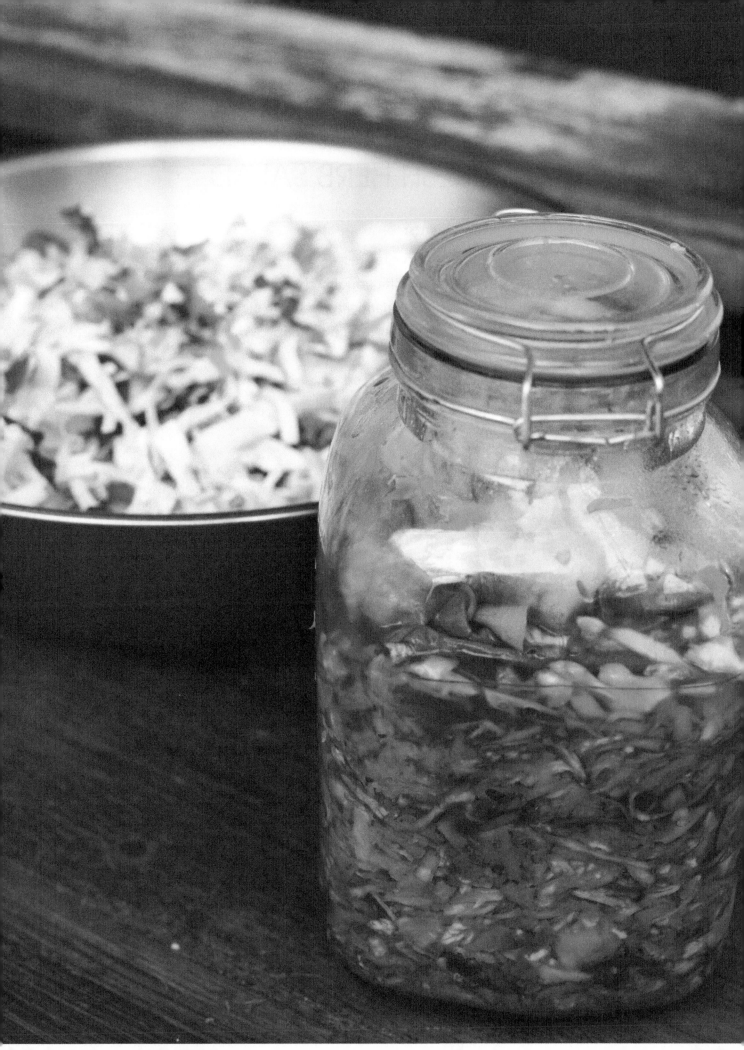

FRESH HERB SALAD

Ingredients:

- 1 bunch of watercress
- 1 bunch of mint (roughly chopped)
- 1 bunch of coriander (picked into pieces; not chopped)
- 1 bunch of basil (roughly chopped)
- Toasted Pepitas
- Toasted sesame seed
- Approx. 150ml of olive oil
- ½ tbsp. of Dijon mustard
- Juice of 1 lemon.

Jo's tips: Be creative and use whatever fresh seasonal herbs that look good. When storing herbs, they will last without wilting for up to a week in the fridge if you wrap them in a few newspaper pages, kitchen papers or a tea towel, and keep the towel or paper damp.

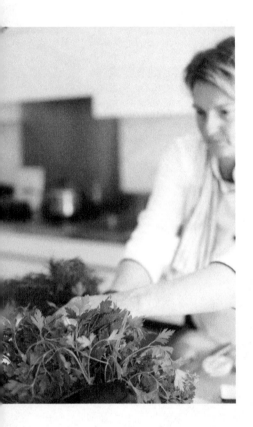

Method:

Combine all herbs in a large bowl.

Mix olive oil, mustard, and lemon juice together (add more or less oil according to how flavoured you like the lemon).

Pour over salad little at a time. You want the salad lightly coated.

Toss through the sesame seed and pepitas.

SPROUTED GREEN SALAD WITH TOASTED SESAME SEEDS

Ingredients:

- 2 handfuls each of lambs lettuce and sunflower sprouts
- 1 handful each of alfalfa sprouts and snow pea sprouts
- 1 cup each of sprouted mung beans, blanched asparagus (sliced), chopped avocado and chopped parsley
- ¾ cup of cherry tomatoes (sliced vertically)
- ½ cup of mixed sesame seeds and sunflower seeds
- 2 tbsp. of organic cold pressed sesame seed oil or flaxseed oil
- ½ lemon (juiced)
- 1 tbsp. of balsamic vinegar
- Pinch of Celtic sea salt.

Method:

Combine lettuce, sprouts, beans, asparagus, parsley and salt together.

Combine oil, lemon juice and balsamic together and fold into salad mix (be gentle and light in your handling).

Sprinkle with mixed seeds and serve.

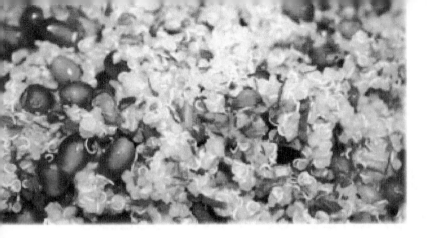

HERBED QUINOA SALAD

Ingredients:

- 2½ cups of vegetable stock or chicken broth
- 1½ cups of quinoa (soak until sprouted, rinse well)
- Celtic sea salt to taste
- 3 tbsp. of chopped fresh herbs (have fun with combining your favourites)
- 2 tsp. of cultured butter.

Jo's tips: Extras that can be added to make a more substantial salad are: cherry tomatoes, pomegranate, sliced celery, and chopped cucumber.

Method:

In a medium saucepan, bring stock to a boil.

Add quinoa, and salt if desired. Reduce heat to low. Cover and cook until quinoa is tender and liquid is absorbed (about 15 minutes).

Remove from heat, add chopped herbs and butter, and serve warm.

SUMMER SALAD

Roast Pumpkin, Beetroot and Walnut salad

Ingredients:

- 1 bag of Baby spinach
- 1 avocado chunky
- ¼ pumpkin chunky
- 4 baby beetroots
- 100g activated walnuts
- 6 grape tomatoes
- 1 tbsp. of organic olive oil
- Dash of balsamic (aged is best)
- 1 tsp. each of ground cumin and coriander
- Celtic sea salt
- Ground black pepper.

Jo's tips: I also love this salad with toasted sesame seeds instead of walnuts, and then using sesame seed oil instead of olive oil.

Method:

Mix pumpkin and baby beetroots with sea salt, pepper, cumin, coriander and a little of the olive oil (about 1tsp.) and roast on baking paper in hot oven for 25 minutes (160°C).

Cool slightly. Gently mix with rest of the ingredients and serve.

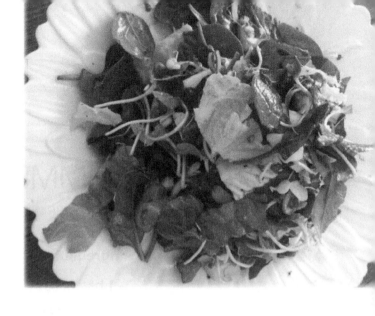

SPRING SALAD

Ingredients:

- 1 Cos Lettuce
- 1 butter lettuce
- 1 packet of sunflower sprouts
- 1 packet of broccoli sprouts
- 1 packet of radish sprouts
- 1 banana (diced)
- ½ punnet cherry tomatoes (halved)
- 1 avocado (diced)
- 50g of toasted coconut.

Jo's tip: Another quality cold pressed oil is flaxseed oil, which is the only polyunsaturated oil I use sparingly. None of the others get a look in. With the way and method they are produced and stored, I consider them to be highly unstable, rancid oils.

DRESSING:

Blend together;

- Juice of 1 lemon
- 3 tbsp. of olive oil
- Salt and pepper to taste.

Gently blend all the ingredients together, add dressing and gently blend again. Top with toasted coconuts and serve.

➜ **Watch it on YouTube** ⬅

Please scan this QR code with your iphone to watch the you tube demonstration of preparing this Summer Salad

PEAR AND PERSIAN GOATS CHEESE SALAD

Ingredients:

- 1 pear (thinly sliced)
- 50g of Persian goats cheese (cut in cubes)
- 15g of crispy walnuts
- Mixed Baby spinach and Rocket
- 1 tbsp. of olive oil
- Juice of ½ lemon
- Celtic sea salt.

Method:

Combine spinach, rocket, walnuts and pear into bowl. Combine the olive oil and lemon juice with salt and pepper. Gently mix through salad and arrange on plate. Arrange goat cheese pieces over and around garish with a couple of extra walnuts.

SWEET TREATS

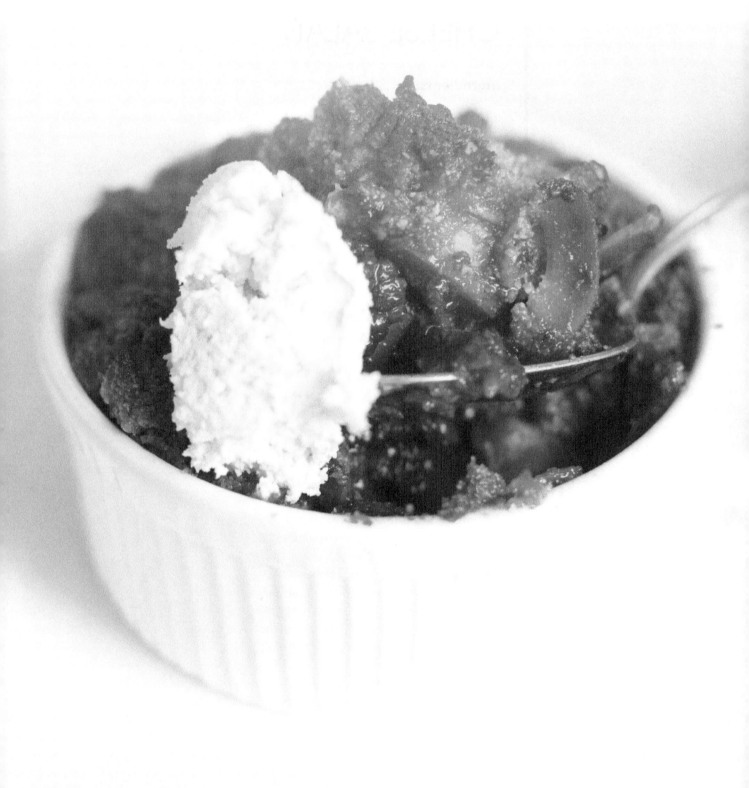

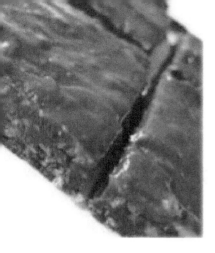

RAW DATES AND ALMOND SLICE

Serves 20 pieces @ $0.75 per serve

Ingredients:

- 1 cup of almonds soaked overnight (discard water)
- 2 cups of dates soaked for couple of hours (1 cup for topping)
- 1 cup of filtered water
- ½ cup of cocoa powder
- 2 cups of chopped coconut meat or desiccated coconut.

Method:

Blend until smooth (almonds, 1 cup of dates and filtered water and carob).

Mix in coconut and press into biscuit tray to about 1 inch in thickness.

Leave covered in fridge for 2 - 3 hours to firm up.

For topping; process the second cup of dates in blender with a little water until smooth like 'cake icing' and spread over the set mix.

Sprinkle with some coconut or other nuts of your choice. Rest in fridge, then cut into squares.

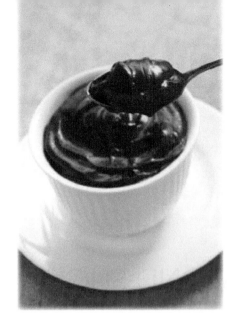

CHOCOLATE MOUSSE

Serves four @ $1.65 per serve

Ingredients:

- 6 pitted fresh dates (soaked and pitted)
- ¼ cup of pure maple syrup or raw honey
- ½ tsp. of vanilla extract
- 2 avocados (mashed)
- ¼ cup of raw organic cocoa powder
- 1 tbsp. of liquid from the soaked dates
- 4 tsp. of toasted coconut flakes to garnish.

Jo's tips: This is a rich, smooth sweet treat! You only need about 2 tbsp. per serve.

If you are sensitive to the caffeine in cocoa, then try substituting with carob powder that is caffeine free.

Method:

Blend dates, maple syrup and vanilla in food processor until smooth.

Add avocado and cocoa powder; process until creamy. Add the date liquid and process briefly.

Divide the mousse between 4 ramekins or tall dessert glasses.

Store in a sealed container.

Mousse will keep for 3 days in a fridge, or 2 weeks in a freezer.

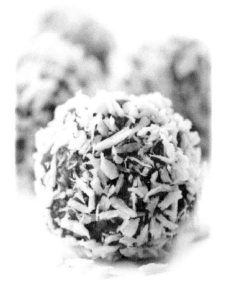

BANNANA AND COCOA BALLS

Makes 24 pieces @ $0.45 per piece

Ingredients:

- 2 bananas
- ½ cup of raw almonds soaked in filtered water overnight or 1 cup of almond meal
- 2 tbsp. of cocoa, or carob powder if sensitive to caffeine
- ½ cup of currants
- ⅓ cup of caramelised buckwheat (optional)
- ½ tsp. of balsamic vinegar
- Desiccated coconut for rolling.

Method:

Drain and process soaked almonds in food processor before adding the rest of the ingredients.

If using almond meal, simply blend bananas, currants, cocoa and vinegar first, and then place mixture in a bowl and add almond meal until mixture is firm enough to roll.

Roll balls in desiccated coconut and place in fridge to firm before serving.

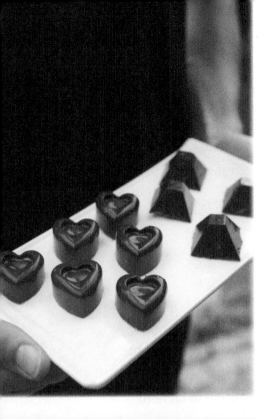

RAW CHOCOLATE

Makes 24 pieces @ $0.35 each

Ingredients:

- 1 ½ cups of cocoa butter
- ½ cup of coconut oil
- ¼ cup of honey, or maple syrup
- 3.5 tbsp. of cocoa powder
- Pinch of Himalayan salt crystals.

Jo's tips: Be creative. Try adding your favourite nuts, dried fruit, a shot of espresso, or another natural essence.

Method:

Melt cocoa butter and coconut oil in a stainless steel bowl over simmering water (not too hot) whisk in your choice of sweetener and blend till until smooth. Add cocoa powder and combine until smooth

Gently pour into moulds and place in fridge to set.

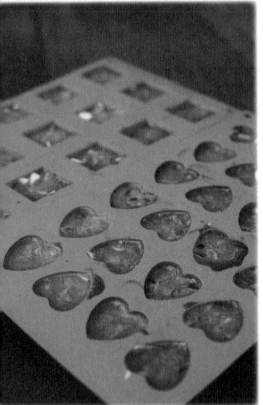

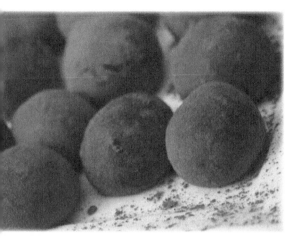

CHOCOLATE BALL

Makes 24 pieces @ $0.35 each

Ingredients:

- 1 ½ cups of cocoa butter
- ½ cup of coconut oil
- ¼ cup of honey, or maple syrup
- 3.5 tbsp. of cocoa powder
- 1/2 cup of coconut flour
- 1 cup of almond meal
- Pinch of Himalayan salt crystals.

Jo's tips: You can create your own variation of chocolate balls once you have made the basic recipe. Perhaps Rum and raisin, mixed nuts, or Goji berries.

Method:

As with the basic chocolate recipe above melt and combine cocoa butter, coconut oil cocoa powder and your choice of sweetener into a blender and blend till until smooth.

Gradually add coconut flour and almond meal. Check taste and add more cocoa powder if needed. The amount of flour and almond meal may vary depending on how wet or dry you want the consistency of your balls to be

Roll into balls, and then roll balls in cocoa powder or shredded coconut.

Store in a sealed container in the fridge.

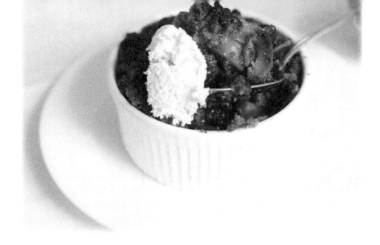

APPLE AND BLUEBERRY CRUMBLE

Serves four @ $2.25 per serve

Ingredients:

- ½ cup of dry coconut flakes
- 1 cup of almond meal
- 4 medium green apples (cored but leave skin on)
- 1 cup of blueberries
- ½ tsp. of vanilla powder
- 3 tbsp. of cold pressed coconut oil or butter
- Aromatic spices such as cloves, nutmeg or cinnamon (½ tsp. each)

Method:

To make the crumble topping, rub the coconut oil or butter into the almond meal and dried coconut flakes, add vanilla and set aside.

Quarter green apples and poach in a small amount of water and aromatic spices with berries, then place in a shallow dish or individual ramekins.

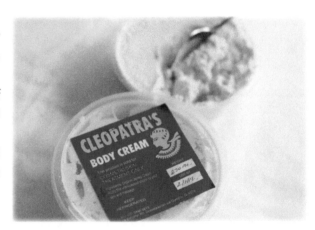

Spread coconut mixture over the top of apples and berries, and bake in the oven at 120ºC until top is golden brown.

Serve with Cleopatra's cream.

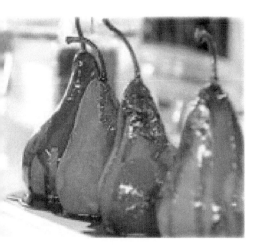

SLOW-COOKED SPICED PEARS

Serves six @ $3.10 per serve

Ingredients:

- 1½ cups of dry red wine
- ½ cup of marsala
- 2 star anise
- 6 medium pears peeled and left whole with stalks intact
- 3 thick strips of lemon rind.

Method:

Combine all the ingredients in the slow cooker and let pears soak for an hour in the liquid mix, while you turn them occasionally to coat evenly.

Cook on low heat for 4 - 6 hours, turning occasionally to coat.

To serve, remove pears from the slow cooker and place onto a serving plate. Pour syrup over pears. Serve with Cleopatra's cream.

ORANGE AND ALMOND CAKE (Gluten free)

Serves eight @ $2.75 per serve

Ingredients:

- 6 eggs
- 250g of ground almonds
- 2 oranges
- 150g of honey
- 1 tsp. of ground cardamom
- 1 tbsp. of baking powder.

Jo's tips: This is one of the moistest cakes I've yet to come up with. There is so much you could try using ½ coconut flour and half almond or hazelnut meal instead, and it would still retain its moisture. The only difference is that it's going to be a little heavier in texture.

Method:

Boil whole oranges for 1 hour, changing water twice to remove bitterness, drain, and cool.

Blend whole oranges in food processor.

Beat eggs, honey and cardamom until creamy, and then stir in the orange pulp.

Add almond meal mixed with baking powder, the mix will be fairly soft. Pour into square or round baking tin and bake at 160°C for 20 - 30 minutes. Check that the batter is cooked with a skewer.

Cool before lifting out and cutting.

CHAPTER 4

WHAT YOU NEED TO KNOW

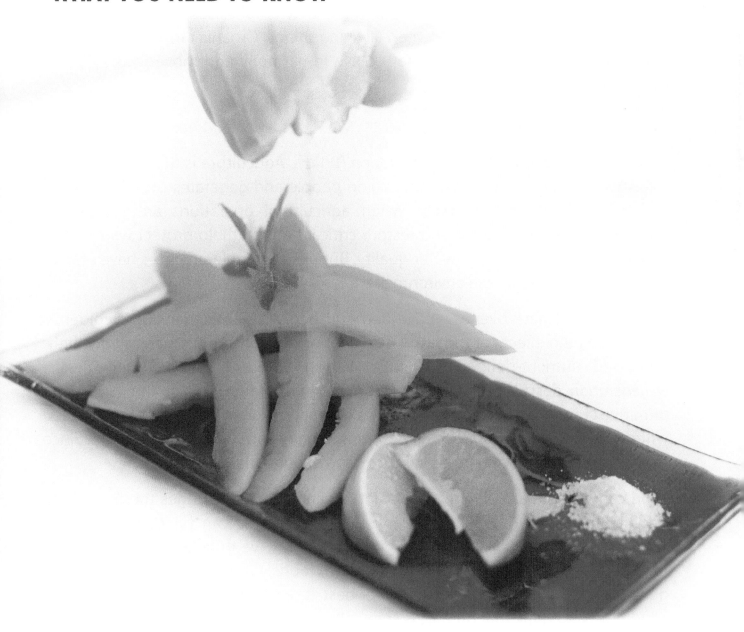

Organic farming is a method of farming that emphasises and promotes the relationships that exist between all living things. Organic farming encourages bio-diversity, where all things in nature live in harmony and move to the natural rhythm and cycles of life.

WHY BUY ORGANIC

According to the *World Wildlife Foundation (WWF)*, "Agriculture is the world's largest industry. It employs more than one billion people and generates over $1.3 trillion dollars worth of food annually. When agricultural operations are sustainably managed, they can preserve and restore critical habitats, help protect watersheds, and improve soil health and water quality. But unsustainable practices have serious impacts on people and the environment."

We are a nation that is over-fed and undernourished. We are experiencing in epidemic proportions the effects of the last 4+ generations of consuming increasingly high-processed, nutrient-deficient foods. Dr. Weston A Price, in *Nutrition and Physical Degeneration* described the introduction of white man's food in the 1930s into primitive cultures as "the displacing foods of modern commerce", namely processed white sugar, processed white flour, pasteurised dairy and processed white salt. Since then, the list of displacing foods has increased exponentially.

Food can be both a problem and a solution, and nutrition bridges the gap where traditional medicine falls short. Many health problems can be corrected or, at least, greatly alleviated, simply by changing the way we think about and relate to food. Choosing LHI (Low Human Intervention) foods, naturally grown and nutrient dense, is leveraging Mother Nature at her best. It saddens me that we have become conditioned to think that organic is some alternative, trendy or hip choice from the "norm", when 100 years ago all food was organic, sourced locally and seasonal. People ate *real* food, prepared and preserved in order to optimise its nutrient value, not to denature it.

Now as a result, many people think the word 'organic' is covert for too expensive or worst still, for hippies! But the fact is more and more people want to eat organically but struggle to adjust their budget to benefit from the long-term gains. We are so conditioned to wanting and expecting instant gratification especially where spending money is concerned. Unless we finally realise that the lifestyle we all aspire to enjoy is really dependent on our and our family's health, chances are the materialistic world of instant pleasure will always take precedence over making choices that support our long-term health.

Eating to stay healthy during the current economic climate doesn't have to send you broke. Neither do you have to take an all-or-nothing approach in order to obtain the benefits of eating organically. Taking a step-by-step approach is a far less stressful and more affordable way to transition.

You don't have to be a rocket scientist these days to realise that there just isn't the same level of nutrient value in our foods that there was 80 years ago. The World Health Organization (WHO) statistics show us that we are a nation with more sickness and disease than we have seen in the last 60 years.

43 million children worldwide under the age of 5 are obese.

2 in every 3 people are at risk of cancer.

Cardiovascular diseases (CVDs) are still the number one cause of death globally.

An estimated 17.3 million people died from CVDs in 2008, representing 30% of all global deaths.

By 2030, it is estimated almost 25 million people will die from CVDs, mainly from heart disease and stroke.

We have more qualified scientists, researchers, doctors, specialists and the most advanced technology ever used, yet we still haven't managed to reverse the diseases that plague our modern lifestyle. And in truth, addressing key risk factors such as unhealthy diets and physical inactivity can prevent most cardiovascular diseases.

During the time of this writing, the first ever, long-term GMO toxicity study was released in September 2012 by French scientist Professor Seralini and his team. A two-year study on feeding rats with genetically modified corn sprayed with a commonly used weedkiller, produced by *Monsanto*, called Roundup (a technology introduced into our food supply in the last 15 years), found tumours and multiple organ damage in these rats. The alarming truth behind the dangers of GMO foods for which we are the guinea pigs is finally here, released in perfect timing as the State of California is lobbying for all GMO foods to be labelled. You can watch a summary of the study on www.youtube.com/watch?v=eeW5yUSqdhY

In the same month, *The Wall Street Journal* reported that Russia's consumer-rights watchdog said it had suspended the import and use of a genetically engineered corn made by *Monsanto Co.* following a study's findings that the suggested crop might cause cancer.

The Institute of Responsible Technologies also released the ground-breaking documentary *Genetic Roulette*, the dangers of GMO foods by Jeffery M. Smith. You can view this documentary at GeneticRouletteMovie.com

Since 1930, we have added in excess of 140,000 new chemicals, not previously in existence, into the environment. Every year, at least 1,500 new chemicals of which many are not tested for toxicity, are added. According to the WWF, the use of pesticides and fertilisers on farms has increased 26 fold over the past 50 years.

We now add chemical preservatives, additives, flavourings, colourings, sweeteners, emulsifiers and stabilisers to our food. We use chemical fertilisers, pesticides, herbicides and fungicides and spray poisons on our produce while it's still growing. We pick it before it's ripe, store it too long, transport it too far, then gas, freeze, irradiate, can, or package it. We are more concerned with how our food looks than how it tastes, and we rarely question its nutrient value and where, when or how it was grown. We are seduced by convenience, marketing and packaging.

Just because this has become the norm in today's food culture doesn't mean it is right. According to Dr. Candice Peart, a world renowned leader in the study and science of the mind-body connection, in her book *Molecules of Emotion, she* states, "as little as 5% of all disease can be attributed to inherited genetics." We are ingrained to think that heart disease, cancer, obesity and diabetes is something that is genetically passed on if you have a family history of it. However, we now know through the science of epigenetics that nutrition, our environment and even our thoughts directly influence our genes and the genetic potential of our children and even their offspring. Perhaps what we actually need to look closely at are the inherited food choices, eating habits and lifestyle factors passed down through generations.

In the last five years, I have seen the food revolution movement gain traction with documentaries such as *Food Inc*, *Sweet Misery*, *The Cure*, *Food Matters* and just recently, *Hungry 4 Change*. We are not lacking information or scientific evidence that conclusively suggests that the only way we can turn these health crises around is by voting with our dollar and taking the responsibility for our health back into our own hands.

I do believe a new consciousness is among us, one that seeks to get back to the source, to find the real food behind what has been processed and manipulated beyond all reason. Ancient and primitive cultures understood food to be sacramental - a sacred offering in which we experience the mystical inter-connectedness of all life; a gift of grace from which we receive the innate intelligence held within the micro-environment whether land or sea, from which that food source originated.

It is this intelligence that our DNA innately knows how to work with to support the optimal expression of our genes. It can be said, quite simply, that the further away our food processing takes us from its original source, the less intelligence our food holds. We are essentially short-changing ourselves by not enabling our bodies to access, on a cellular level, the vital information that they need in order to repair and regenerate themselves to their original health and vital expression.

In a nutshell, if the food wasn't around when your great grandmother was alive, don't eat it!

12 REASONS TO BUY ORGANIC

1. **Organic food is better for your health:** There is compelling research that shows that organic food is far superior in its nutrient value with up to 40% more nutrients than commercially farmed foods. Organic food is also richer in vital secondary nutrients such as vitamins, minerals, trace mineral and enzymes especially vitamin C, iron, magnesium, calcium, and phosphorus. These secondary nutrients are vital in order for the body to break down the fats, proteins and carbohydrates and making them bio-available to the body. Believe it or not, when you are consistently eating nutrient-dense foods, you actually begin to eat less, as your body not only feels satisfied but also nourished, and therefore doesn't constantly crave more food, which is often the case with denatured and nutrient-deficient foods.

2. **Organic food is rocket fuel:** Organic food has more life force (energy) due to its superior electromagnetic nutrients held in the soils and plants. This means you will have a whole lot more energy to do a whole lots more of what you love!

3. **You can actually make money:** Because time is money and you will have more energy you will be more productive in achieving so much more in the same amount of time as you did before, which will increase your earning potential experientially.

4. **Organic farming is more energy efficient:** Organic farming methods use less fuel than conventional farming which uses more petroleum than most other industries, not to mention their blueprint due to the production of synthetic fertilisers, pesticides, herbicides and fungicides.

5. **Organic food tastes better:** I know I'm a chef and therefore flavour is everything, but seriously, organic just downright tastes better!

6. **Organic farming methods help to protect future generations:** Organic farming starts with the nourishment of the soil. There is up to 85% more micro-organisms in organic soil, which leads to the nourishment of plants and animals and ultimately, the nourishment of our bodies. The average child receives approximately four times more exposure than an adult to a number of widely used cancer-causing pesticides in food. Children under six years of age are at higher risk because of their body composition. Until age six, their body is made up of more water and less fat than adults. This means they are less able to 'trap' and store chemical toxins in fatty tissue. The food choices we make now determine our children's health not only now but also in the future.

7. **Certified organic means GMO free:** Genetically modified organisms are strictly not allowed under organic certification standards.

8. **Certified organic foods are not irradiated:** Food irradiation is a process of exposing fresh and packaged food to ionising radiation to destroy micro-organisms, bacteria, viruses or insects that might be present in the food. Unfortunately, the process also kills all known nutrient value of the food as well. Currently, there is no legislation enforcing the labelling of irradiated foods in Australia.

9. **Certified organic food is free of artificial chemicals, hormones and antibiotics:** Organic food does not contain food additives, preservatives, artificial colouring, emulsifiers, stabilisers or the use of antibiotics, anti-microbials, recombinant bovine growth hormone (rBGH), all of which can cause health problems such as heart diseases, tumours, osteoporosis, birth deformities and cancer. In the case where livestock are treated with veterinary drugs or chemicals, they are prohibited from being sold as organic.

10. **Support your local farmers:** When we purchase organic food we support traditional farming methods. Most organic farms are small, independent, family-owned farms of less than 100 hectares. Many family farms have been to sell-up since the industrial age of agro farming monopolised the economic market.

11. **Living in harmony with nature:** When Mother Nature is allowed to exist within a natural, organic, closed chain cycle, our plants, oceans and waterways aren't

polluted. Environmental toxins are minimised and plants, animals and man thrive.

12. **You can actually save money:** When you decide that you're worth the investment and start to eat organically whenever possible, you will notice a saving made on money spent on doctor's visits, vitamin and mineral supplements, drug prescriptions and medications. We have been eating organically as a family for the last four years and I haven't had the flu nor been taken out by a cold or infection in this time. My immune system is twice as strong as it has ever been. This is undecidedly one of the best investments you could make for your future health.

> *Paving the way for a healthier future is as much about looking after one's self as it is about looking after the next generations that follow our example.*

ORGANIC CERTIFICATION STANDARDS

There are many different private certification bodies that claim to be a guide for what is and isn't healthy. The Heart Foundation of Australia's Tick √ is a good example. There is still a percentage of the Australian population that actively seek out products that have this Tick symbol as reassurance that that food is healthy. But it's more complicated than that: The Tick indicates a product is healthier than other options, but it doesn't mean it's healthy in its own right. For manufacturers to be awarded the Heart Foundation Tick, they have to demonstrate that the product meets nutritional standards. However, no standards are set to demonstrate the source or quality of the nutrients. Where a food comes from and how it is processed determines, not just it's nutrient value but, more importantly, the quality of its nutrients. In September 2011, the Heart Foundation announced plans to revoke its Tick from fast food takeaway outlets. I believe this speaks a thousand words about the credibility of this symbol.

The same caution needs to be taken when sourcing organically. Please do not just assume that if a product is labelled organic or has the word 'organic' written somewhere on the packaging, that it is (a) certified organic or that (b) it is healthy.

How do we know if a product is really organic?

Wikipedia's definition of organic is 'a matter that has come from a once-living organism, is capable of decay or the product of decay, or is composed of organic compound containing carbon.' This makes it pretty hard not to name most things in life organic, which is why it gives marketing executives license to have a field day when labelling their products 'organic' all too often at our expense.

117

For a product to be certified organic, it has to contain a minimum of 95% organically produced ingredients. The remaining 5% has to be made from non-synthetic natural ingredients. For the consumer to be sure that the product is actually organic, it needs to be certified as organic.

ORGANIC CERTIFICATION AGENCIES IN AUSTRALIA

There are seven independent certification agencies in Australia that meet the Australian Certified Organic Standards (ACOS) that:

1. Improve the structure, fertility, and health of the soil while enhancing the surrounding environment. Artificial fertilisers, pesticides and herbicides and fungicides are prohibited

2. Produce quality agricultural and livestock products, true to species, with high nutritional value. GMOs are strictly prohibited at every stage of production. GMOs are not allowed on the same production unit, even if you are not seeking certification of that area.

3. Avoid pollution resulting from agriculture

4. Minimise the use of non-renewable resources

5. Increase biodiversity

6. Work towards being a closed system

For a complete guide to the AOS, please visit http://www.bfa.com.au

Australia's 7 Certification agencies are:

- Australian Certified Organic Pty Ltd. (ACO)

- The National Association for Sustainable Agriculture, Australia (NASAA)

- AUS – QUAL Pty Ltd., a subsidiary to the Australian Meat Industry Standards and Quality System Management Company

- Australian Growers Association (AGO)

- Organic Food Chain Pty Ltd. (OFC)

- Tasmanian Organic-Dynamic Producers (TOP)

- The Bio-dynamic research institute is the Australian certification body for DEMETER biodynamic methods. Biodynamic production systems are based on principles established by Dr. Rudolph Steiner in 1924.

For a global reference, The Organic Certification Directory 2012 can be sourced from http://www.organicstandards.com

GUIDELINES WHEN BUYING NON-CERTIFIED ORGANIC PRODUCE

Understanding additional labelling:

Free-range: This label indicates that the flock was provided shelter in a building, room or area with unlimited access to food, fresh water, and continuous access to the outdoors during their production cycle. The label does not reflect or regulate the use of chemicals, antibiotics, hormones, pesticides or the quality of the feed provided.

Cage-free: This label indicates that the flock was able to freely roam a building, room or enclosed area with unlimited access to food and fresh water during their production cycle. The label does not reflect or regulate the use of chemicals, antibiotics, hormones, pesticides or the quality of the feed provided.

Natural: Don't be fooled by labels that claim to be natural. Only meat, poultry, and egg products labelled as natural must be minimally processed and contain no artificial ingredients. However, the natural label does not include any standards regarding farm practices or use of chemicals, antibiotics, hormones, pesticides or the quality of the feed provided and only applies to the processing of meat and egg products. Further more there are no standards or regulations for the labelling of 'natural' food products if they do not contain meat or eggs.

Grass-fed: Grass-fed animals receive a majority of their nutrients from grass throughout their life, while an organic animal's pasture diet may be supplemented with organic grain. The grass-fed label does not limit the use of antibiotics, hormones, or pesticides. Meat products may be labelled as grass-fed organic.

If you are having a month where you just can't afford certified organic products, then the following produce guidelines will help you choose the healthiest alternatives:

Reference the following choices when certified organic isn't possible

Meat, Poultry and Eggs:

- Locally farmed
- Pasture or grass fed, chemical and hormone free
- Free range
- Cage-free.

Dairy:

- Grass-fed
- Full fat
- Un-homogenised
- Unfortified.

Fruit and Vegetables:

- Locally grown
- Pesticide and chemical free.

CHAPTER 5

MAKING EVERY MOUTHFUL COUNT

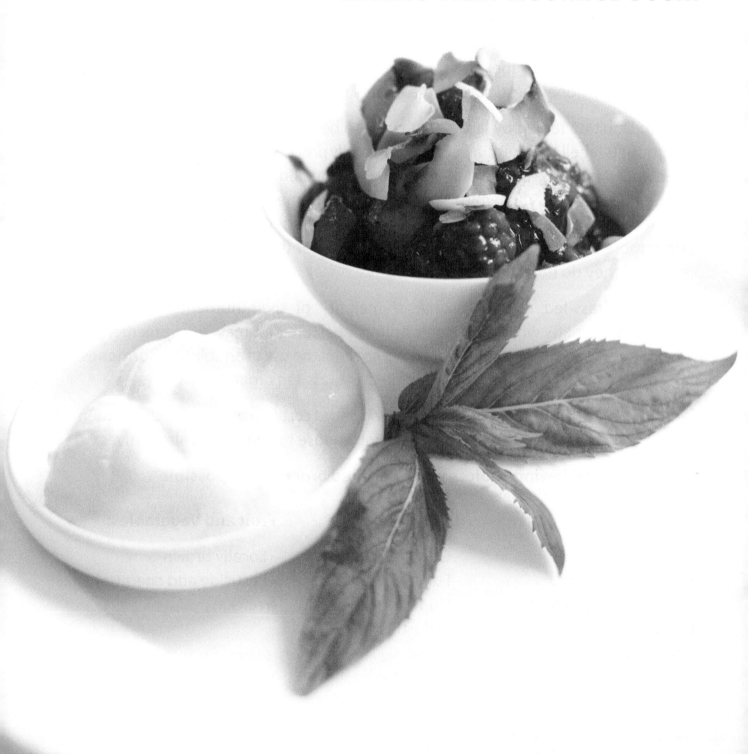

I believe that the single most important thing you can do when trying to get healthy without going broke is to know that you are getting bang for your buck and making every mouthful count. Knowing where and how your product has been raised and produced is vital in the quest for optimal and sustainable health and vitality. You need to know your product is KING - the very best *your* money can buy.

Reference the following guidelines when deciding on where to buy from:

Local and seasonal is always the best

Foods grown in sync with the seasons are more in tune with our intuitive nutritional needs. We also save on import and transport costs.

Organic straight from the farm

If you want to be sure that you are getting full value for your money, then buy directly from the farm. My family and I live in the hub of Sydney, yet we still manage to source our meats either straight from the farmer or a butcher we know and trust. It may require a little extra time and research but the return on your investment will save you money in the long term.

Organic farmers markets

These are a great way to support your local farming community and save on the middleman costs. Be mindful however that there are going to be growers that aren't organic so don't assume anything. Also watch for the promoters of 'natural'; look closely and ask questions because as often as not, their food can just be processed rubbish.

Your Local Organic Grocer or Co-op

They usually have a good reputation for supporting local produce with minimal organic imports. Great place to purchase whole foods in bulk.

Organic Online / home delivery

There are some great online organic home delivery services and, depending on your location, delivery can be free. This method of purchasing has its residual benefits saving on money, travel time and petrol.

Supermarket Organics

Coles and Woolworths now control around 80% of our food chain and import over 50% of our food from overseas including its organic offerings. Buying organic from these monopoly supermarkets dilute the very intent of 'organic' since *much of their organic produce are shipped in from around the world, carrying no sense of connection with its geography or its farmers.*

Today, it's common to think of food as a predominate source of energy or fuel for the body. We're taught to count calories and either cut or increase them as needed, following a 'one-fits-all' approach to weight control. Many of my clients, when they start working with me, have very little understanding of where or how their food is sourced and even less knowledge of its nutritional value. As a result, many are nutritionally deficient and adopt the 'vitamins and supplementation will save me' attitude, believing that they can make up for a diet that lacks the full spectrum of nutrients needed by taking a multivitamin tablet. Sorry, but that's just not possible.

It's important not to confuse a food's life force or intelligence with its caloric value or with its nutrimental value in protein, fats or carbohydrates. The life force of a food is dependent on the presence of actively available co-factors such as enzymes, vitamins, minerals, trace minerals and beneficial bacteria. Without these elements, the body will be unable to breakdown, digest and absorb the benefits of the proteins, fats and carbohydrates. These essential co-factors are produced in the soil by the alchemic relationship between organic matter and micro-organisms.

Modern farming methods of today have significantly reduced the levels of micro-organisms and organic matter, leaving our soils devoid of the essential elements from which the plant kingdom draws its nutrients and intelligent life force. The animal kingdom becomes a rich and condensed source of nutrients when the animals graze on organic pastures. However, non-organic soils have up to 85% less micro-organism life than organic soils, leaving our plants and animals lacking these essential nutrients.

TOP 12 TIPS FOR SAVING MONEY ON ORGANIC PRODUCE

1. Avoid impulse purchases

When you don't have a shopping list, you are susceptible to impulse buying and spending money on items that really aren't of benefit. Always plan your meals ahead of time. Do a 'pantry stock take' before referring to your meal plans for specific ingredients and amounts required.

2. Eat before you shop

Shopping when you're hungry will eat into your budget. We have all experienced the effects of freshly baked goods and other mouth-watering aromas that can weaken the hardiest of shoppers.

3. Grocery store loyalty program / coupons

Find out what food coupon or discount offer your local organic grocer offers. At ours, you get a $5 gift voucher for every $100 you spend. This is redeemable against supplements and household cleaning products or personal items. We save these every week and are able to buy all our organic shampoos once a month for FREE!

4. Buy in bulk

This is a great way to save money on the whole food dry goods like whole grains, legumes, beans, pulses, nuts and seeds that have a longer shelf life. These can often be purchased at great bulk prices at your local organic co-op.

When we buy in bulk fresh organic meat in our household, we buy a whole biodynamic lamb straight from the farm for $210. We choose the cuts and portion sizes we want and they vacuum pack, ready for the freezer. Sometimes we share the cost with another family and it is a great way to get the biggest bang for your buck, not to mention the peace of mind that you will have that your purchases are of the BEST quality.

5. Join a co –op

By becoming a member and supporting your local organic co–op, you can get up to 10% - 15% off the non-member retail price.

6. Shop seasonally

Supply and demand always keeps costs down and when you are buying what is seasonally available to your area, you won't be paying premium prices for foods that are imported because they aren't in season.

7. Shop locally

Support your local growers and suppliers. There are no import costs, or transportation and storage costs when you buy locally.

8. Buy unprocessed foods

When you make the choice to stick to fresh produce only, not only is it healthier, but it is cheaper too, because you won't be paying for the processing and packaging.

9. Grow your own

One guaranteed way of saving money on organic food is to grow your own! Keep it simple and manageable and if you're a family it's a wonderful thing to get the kids involved. Even if you don't have a garden, start with an herb garden on your window or balcony.

10. Seek out reduced perishable items

You just need to know where and when to look. All fresh produce is perishable and all supermarkets, even your local organic groceries, have set delivery days for fresh produce. It's always rare that there'll be some leftover items from week to week, so ask them what days they discount any leftover perishables to sell quickly to make room for the next fresh deliveries and make note to shop on that day.

Always look for discounted items and check the used by date.

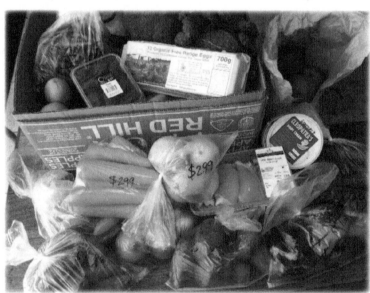

All this and so much more for just **$145**!

11. Shop with cash

You'll never be tempted to overspend if you leave credit and ATM cards at home and bring only enough cash for the food on your shopping list.

12. Stick to the clean 15

The Dirty Dozen and *Clean15* are smart incentives made available by The Environmental Working Group (EWC) who estimates that we can reduce our exposure to pesticides by 80% if we simply know which foods typically have the highest pesticide residue and therefore should only ever be bought if organic. This is great news for us budget-conscious consumers who want to start buying more organically but can't necessarily afford it 100% of the time. The Shopper's Guide to Pesticides in Produce can be found at http://www.ewg.org/foodnews. It will help you determine which fruits and vegetables have the most pesticide residues and therefore are most important to buy organic. In 2012, the EWG included a Plus category to highlight two additional crops in the *Dirty Dozen* category namely - green beans and leafy greens, i.e. kale and spinach - that did not meet traditional *Dirty Dozen* criteria but were commonly contaminated with highly toxic organophosphate insecticides. These insecticides are toxic to the nervous system and have been largely removed from agriculture over the past decade.

The list of *Dirty Dozen plus 2* and the *Clean 15* as of November 2012 are:

Dirty Dozen:

- Apples
- Celery
- Sweet bell peppers (capsicum)
- Strawberries
- Nectarines - Imported
- Grapes
- Spinach
- Lettuce
- Cucumbers
- Blueberries
- Potatoes
- + Kale & greens

Clean 15:

Clean 15 have less pesticide residue and can help when on a budget but I still recommend buying organic whenever possible.

- Onions
- Sweet corn
- Pineapple
- Avocado
- Cabbage
- Sweet pea

- Asparagus

- Mangoes

- Eggplant

- Kiwi

- Cantaloupe (Rockmelon)

- Sweet potato

- Grapefruit

- Watermelon

- Mushrooms

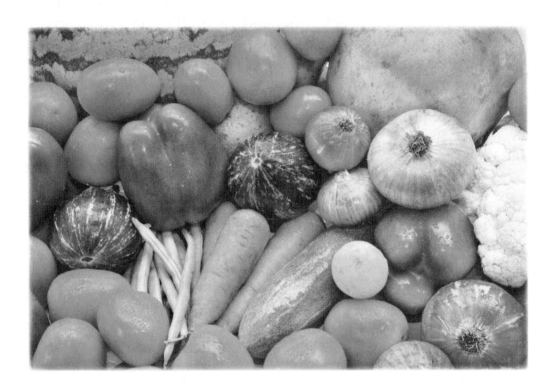

The No. 1 reason that a person goes to see their GP is fatigue, and the most commonly prescribed drug worldwide is an anti–inflammatory, both of which can be either reversed or significantly reduced by eating clean whole food in the right balance for your biochemical and metabolic needs.

CHAPTER 6

31 ACHIEVEABLE TIPS FOR LASTING HEALTH AND VITALITY

1. Learn to listen to your body's wisdom through what it is 'feeling'. It will tell you what it needs at any given moment in time, and often, it's not what you 'think' it needs. Being efficiently able to interpret your body's messages takes practice. For example, when you crave a caffeine or sugar fix, do you really think that your body would tell you it needs a coffee or a coke? Don't you think it could be that your body is trying to communicate to you that it is in need of some 'real' food and water to balance blood sugar levels and replenish and sustain its energy levels?

2. Don't skip breakfast. Missing just one meal increases the release of lipogenic (fat storing) enzymes which subsequently decreases the desired lipolytic (fat burning) enzymes, as researched by Debra Waterhouse, author of *Out Smarting the Female Fat Cell.*

3. Make sure all meals, including breakfast, have all three major food groups; carbohydrates, protein and fat. Most people start the day with a carbohydrate and/ caffeine fix only. This increases your chances of getting hypoglycemia as it instantly creates insulin and a stress response in your body. All this before your day has even started! Your body has its own unique requirements for how much protein, fat and carbohydrate it needs and you can experiment this using the 21-day meal plan to find out what amount of each food group feels right to have at each meal.

4. If you're challenged with digestive problems, then eat smaller meals more often.

5. Don't watch stressful TV or read stressful material while eating as it elicits a stress response (fight or flight response) in your body that decreases the blood flow and energy supply to your digestive system.

6. Chew your water to exude the most benefit and drink your food. In other words; chew till it's liquefied!

7. Avoid foods that you are intolerant or allergic to. It may sound like an obvious tip but I've lost count of the number of clients who, even when they know they have grain and or dairy intolerance, still choose to eat these foods and then later complain of the consequences. I have seen countless symptoms like fatigue, bloating, joint pain, inflammation, mental fogginess and mild depression drop away by excluding all grains and dairy. With over 300,000 plants and over a million animal species to choose from, don't let the well-what-am-I-supposed-to-eat attitude become the excuse for continued suffering, because you definitely have a choice!

8. Avoid all soy products unless they are organic and fermented using traditional methods of fermentation. Unfermented soybeans contain potent anti-nutrients. In their natural form, soybeans contain phytochemicals that have a toxic effect on the human body. The three major anti-nutrients are phytates, enzyme inhibitors and goitrogens.

9. Always soak all nuts, seeds, pulses, grains and legumes for at least 12 - 24 hours, or until sprouted, if applicable to the product. This will ensure that the phytates are neutralised.

10. Going to sleep by 10 pm and rising by 6 am or with the sun has a positive effect on every system of the body, especially the Hormonal System. Remember that your circadian rhythms are governed by the rising and setting of the sun and the moon. The hormones related to physical growth and repair of the body are secreted between the hours of 10 pm and 2 am. The hormones related to mental and emotional rejuvenation are secreted between the hours of 2 am and 6 am. If we were able to control or manipulate these rhythms, then we wouldn't suffer from the effects associated with sleep deprivation but we can't - ask any mother or shift worker!

11. For a better night's sleep, minimise your exposure to bright lights, especially fluorescent lights, for at least 2 hours before bed. Light stimulates cortisol production that needs to be significantly reduced in order for melatonin (the body's sleep hormone) to be released. If you don't have dimmer switches, use candles or lamps with low wattage light bulbs. Avoid stimulants like a workout, caffeine, sugar, alcohol, and nicotine or action/thriller movie after 2 pm as they all stimulate an increase in cortisol levels.

12. Taking a cold shower for 3 - 6 minutes once a day (anytime of the day) is beneficial. It helps to regulate your adrenal glands and metabolic rate as well as strengthen your immune system. I've been doing them for a few months and my energy levels have substantially increased.

13. Drink adequate amounts of quality water between meals. The ideal amount is based on your body weight. This formula comes from the research by Dr. Batmangheildj in his book, *Your Body's Many Cries for Water*. Calculate 0.003 x kg (your body weight) = the amount in litres you need to be consuming per day, before you take into account exercise or consumed stimulants that dehydrate you like coffee, tea, sugar, alcohol, soft drinks and processed foods.

14. Follow the 21-day meal plan with shopping lists provided in this book. The planning has already been done for you.

15. Rotate your foods. If you love certain foods and don't want to risk creating intolerance to that food through over-indulgence, then rotate that food every four days.

16. Avoid the four white devils: processed flour, sugar, table salt, processed dairy.

17. If you can't pronounce a word on the label don't eat it. Chances are your liver wont like it!

18. Unless naturally preserved, the longer the shelf life the worse it is for you.

19. Consume small amounts of fermented vegetables with each main meal. They are a wonderful natural probiotic; rich in digestive enzymes that aid digestion.

20. Cook once and eat twice. Make double for dinner and take to work for lunch.

21. Invest in a slow cooker; it reduces the time spent prepping and cooking by at least half.

22. Don't get caught short. Always travel with a healthy snack like some raw organic nuts or an apple.

23. Avoid drinking alcohol on an empty stomach. Always have some quality fat like a piece of cheese, some nuts, chicken liver pate or avocado to slow down the insulin response.

24. If the food isn't of the same quality or wasn't around when your great grandmother was alive, don't eat it! Most foods that make up today's staple foods are poorly sourced and highly processed. A good example of this is bread. The bread of 70 years ago was a far superior product than the common white and whole-meal loaf available today and is so nutrient deficient that they had to fortify it with synthetic vitamins and minerals. Laugh when they

try to convince you that this is an added value through clever marketing tricks!

25. Don't sweat the small stuff. By identifying and making a plan to alleviate the chief stressor in your life, you often create a domino effect that substantially reduces other stressors simultaneously. Create short-term goals using the smarter analogy in Chapter 1 that helps you to clearly recognise progress as it is achieved.

26. To "workin" or "workout" is a phrase coined by Paul Chek to question one's readiness to expend energy. We all know the physiological and psychological benefits of exercise. However, 'exercise' in most people's minds means to exert themselves through movement, often at the cost of energy that they don't have in reserve to give. If by working out and expending energy, you do not feel energised but instead feel further depleted of energy following the initial short-lived adrenal high, then this would be a good indication that a "workin" session is what you need. You can still exercise (move your body) in ways that actually cultivate and build the body's *Chi* (energy) supplies by engaging in activities such as restorative yoga, *Tai Chi*, *Qi gong*, walking mediations. The point is to use exercise as a stress management tool to support the cultivation of your health and vitality; not diminish it.

27. Address every fungus and/ parasite infection or you will forever be laden with symptoms that are commonly misdiagnosed and treated inappropriately with prescription drugs that at best elevate symptoms in the short term. I strongly recommend you read *The Fungal Link* by Doug Kaufmann.

28. Avoid the top 15 mistakes people make when trying to get healthy – *see Chapter 1*.

29. Live the 80/20 rule. Fad diets are unsustainable in the long term. If you're making the right choices 80% of the time, your body will bounce back with little argument the 20% of the time you wander off your path. That way, the 20% choice is always a good reminder for why you choose the optimal choices 80% of the time. I mean, seriously, who in their right minds wants to feel tired, sick, bloated, depressed, inflamed, weak and prone to injury 80% of their life!

30. Make time to do more of what you love; it's life affirming.

31. Practice gratitude for all that you are, for all that you have, and all that you wish to become, and share with others. Recent research into *How the New Science of Gratitude Can Make You Happier* (Houghton Mifflin, 2007) is summarised in Robert Emmons' new book *Thanks!*

The research on gratitude confronts the idea of a "set point" for happiness; a belief that, just as our body has a set point for weight, each person may have a genetically-determined level of happiness. The set point concept is supported by research that shows that people return to a characteristic level of happiness a short time after both unusually good and unusually bad events. However, we now know from the science of epigenetics that we can influence our own genetic expression and potential through our thoughts as explained in Bruce Lipton's book *Biology of Belief*. The research on gratitude suggests that people can move their set point upward to some degree, enough to have a measurable effect on both their outlook and their health.

Summarising the findings from studies to date, Emmons said that those who practice grateful thinking "reap emotional, physical and interpersonal benefits." People who regularly keep a gratitude journal report fewer illness symptoms, feel better about their lives as a whole, and are more optimistic about the future. Emmons conclusion is that gratitude is a choice; one possible response to our life experiences.

> *"When diet is wrong, medicine is of no use; when diet is correct medicine is of no need."*
> *- Ancient Ayurvedic Proverb.*

CHAPTER 7

RESOURCES

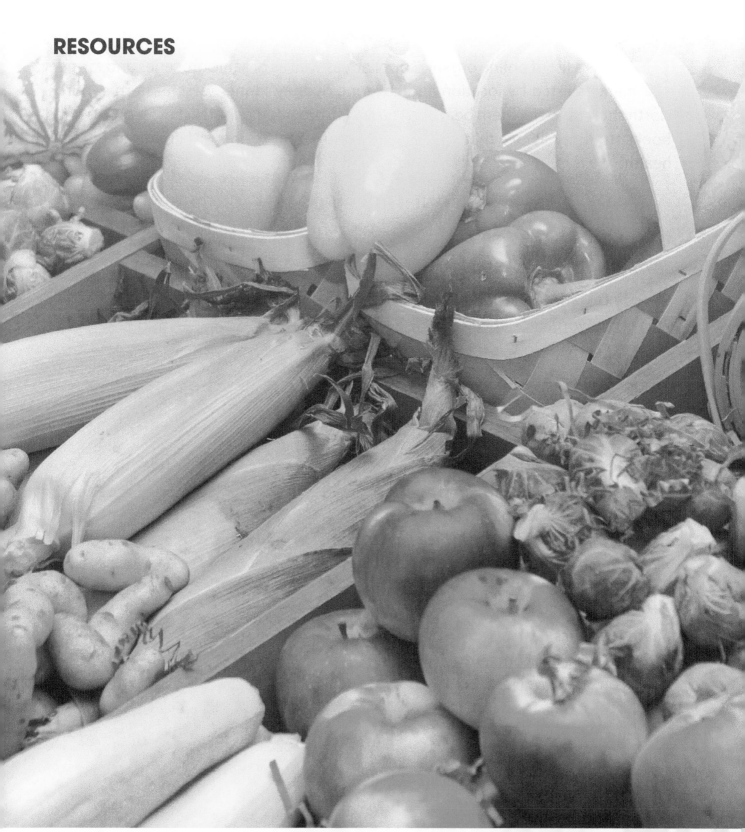

Below is a list of online organic suppliers, as well as organic groceries and farmers markets listed by location and covering Sydney's Inner west, Eastern suburbs, North shore, and Northern beaches. I have also provided a short list of recommended books from my library that have been instrumental to the reclaiming of my own health.

ONLINE SUPPLIERS:

Doorstep Organics
www.doorsteporganics.com.au

Strictly Organic (Meat and Poultry only)
www.strictlyorganic.net.au;
Phone: (02) 43400699.

The Organic Grocer
www.theorganicgrocer.com.au;
Phone: 1300 881171
Email: info@theorganicgrocer.com.au

Moorlands Biodynamic Lamb
www.biodynamiclamb.com.au
(*We love farmer Vince! You can meet him at Everleigh markets. He has a wonderful newsletter too.*)

GROCERS:

Taste Organics
www.tasteorganic.com.au
25 Falcon St, Crows Nest.

About Life

www.aboutlife.com.au/store

Shops: Cammeray: 520 Miller St., Bondi Junction; 31-37 Oxford St. Rozelle; 605 Darling St. Balmain

Ingredients for Health

www.ingredientsforhealth.com.au

132 Willoughby Road Crows Nest NSW 2065

Phone: (02) 9438 3285.

OVViO Organic Health & Lifestyle Store

www.ovvioorganics.com.au

2 Heeley St., Paddington.

For the most incredible organic herbs & spices, teas; of course the wonderful Anthia Koullouros, Naturopath, Herbalist, Health, Food & Lifestyle Educator

Organic Food Network Pty Ltd.

Phone: 02 9938 2364

Fax: 02 9938 2478

E-mail: ofn@bigpond.com

Grass Roots Urban Butchery (GRUB)

www.grassrootsurbanbutchery.com

Vaucluse: 101 New South Head Road (Monday - Friday 7 am – 7 pm; Saturday 7 am – 4 pm)

Phone: (02) 9337 3063

Markets Times and Locations

SUBURB: Chatswood
DAY/TIME: Saturday (8.30 am to 1 pm)
LOCATION: Chatswood Public School, Pacific Highway, Chatswood.

SUBURB: Double Bay
DAY/TIME: Thursday (9.00 am to 2 pm)
LOCATION: Double Bay, Guilfoyle Park, Guilfoyle Avenue, Double Bay.

SUBURB: Frenchs Forest
DAY/TIME: Sunday (8.00 am to 1 pm)
LOCATION: Frenchs Forest, 35 Frenchs Forest Road East, Frenchs Forest.

SUBURB: Gladesville
DAY/TIME: Saturday (9.00 am to 1 pm)
LOCATION: Riverside Girls High School, Cnr Victoria & Huntleys Point Road, Gladesville.

SUBURB: Hornsby
DAY/TIME: Thursday (8.00 am to 4 pm)
LOCATION: Hornsby, Hornsby Mall, Florence Street & Hunter S, Hornsby.

SUBURB: Kings Cross
DAY/TIME: Saturday (8.00 am to 2 pm)
LOCATION: Kings Cross, Fitzroy Gardens, Macleay Street, Kings Cross.

SUBURB: Leichardt
DAY/TIME: Saturday (8.00 am to 1 pm)
LOCATION: Orange Grove Public School, Cnr Perry Street & Balmain Road, Leichhardt.

SUBURB: Marrickville
DAY/TIME: Sunday (8.30 am to 3 pm)
LOCATION: Marrickville, 142 Addison Road, Addison Road Centre, Marrickville.

SUBURB: Newcastle
DAY/TIME: Wednesday to Saturday (9.00 am to 3 pm)
LOCATION: Newcastle, Hunter Street Mall, Hunter Street, Newcastle.

SUBURB: Rouse Hill
DAY/TIME: Saturday (9.00 am to 2 pm)
LOCATION: Rouse Hill Market Sq, Cnr Market Ln and Tempus St , Rouse Hill.

SUBURB: Eveleigh
DAY/TIME: Saturday (8 am – 1 pm)
LOCATION: Carriageworks, 245 Wilson St, Eveleigh.
(Our absolute favourite is Kurrawong Organics; visit Quentin and Leslie Bland).

SUBURB: Pyrmont
DAY/TIME: Saturday (7am-11am)
LOCATION: Piramma Road, Pyrmont.

SUBURB: Fox Studios Entertainment http://www.eqmoorepark.com.au/home/
DAY/TIME: Wed & Sat (10 am - 3.30 pm); Sun (10 am – 4 pm)
LOCATION: Quarter 122 Lang Rd, Moore Park.

SUBURB: Parramatta
DAY/TIME: Saturday (8 am - 1 pm)
LOCATION: Church Street Mall, Parramatta.

When buying organic, foods can be delivered to your door weekly, or you can go direct to the markets to meet the farmers. Ask them what they feed their livestock with, or put into their soil. Fresh is always best!

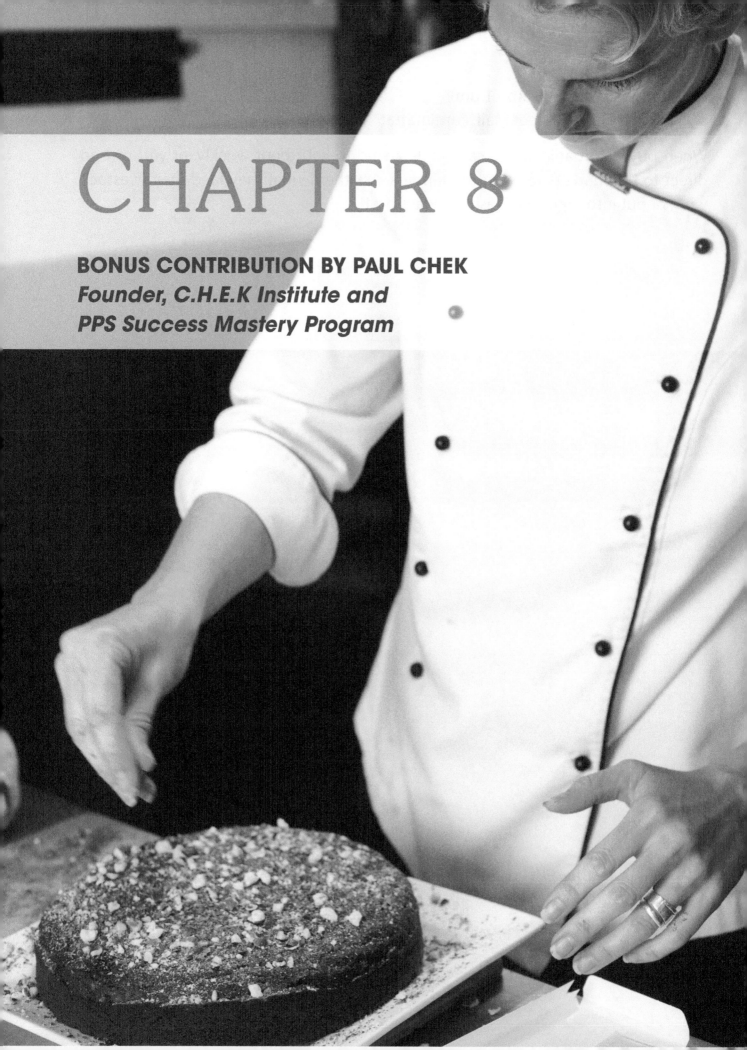

CHAPTER 8

BONUS CONTRIBUTION BY PAUL CHEK
*Founder, C.H.E.K Institute and
PPS Success Mastery Program*

If you want to reach the stars, you will need rocket fuel!

The good news is, the kind of rocket fuel you'll need isn't expensive and is available to you now. The kind of fuel we need to reach the stars (become fully awakened human beings) is exactly what the stars created for us. Without the stars, there would be no planets. Without our sun, there would be no life or food on our own planet.

Though science has gone a long way to create rockets that penetrate the depths of outer space and provide us with beautiful pictures of our galactic home, it hasn't done as well to create beautiful pictures *at home.* When you consider all the food and drug products that have been *scientifically validated,* only to be pulled off shelves later due to significant numbers of people becoming seriously ill or dying from their use, caution is inspired among the wise.

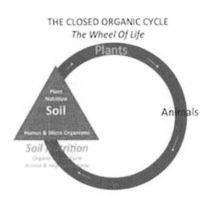

THE CLOSED ORGANIC CYCLE
The Wheel Of Life

As you can see in my diagram, the soil is the foundation of all life. Most people think that *dirt is dead.* The truth is; the soil is never dead *until we kill it.* The same science that makes rocket fuel and munitions was used to create chemical fertilizers and extremely dangerous pesticides, herbicides, fungicides and rodenticides. In the year 1945, it has been estimated that about 200,000 pounds of chemical agents were used on farming soils. Recent estimates suggest that we are now using over 2 BILLION pounds of chemicals on our farmlands. But wait… it gets even more interesting… *crop losses have doubled since 1945!*

If the farming chemicals (also scientifically validated) are working so well, why do commercial farmers need more and more of them every year, while seeing a progressive decline in yields? To answer that question, we need only refer back to a comment made by Sir Albert Howard, still considered today to have been one of (if not) the most eminent agriculturalist of our era. In his writings, Sir Albert Howard informed us that *the bugs always give the farmer his report card.*

To prove his point, Sir Albert Howard grew organic crops and commercial crops. While he was growing the crops, he harvested barrels of plant pests or parasites that were known to feed off the plants he grew. He then exposed the plants to a massive dose of plant pests. He showed that crop losses were only about 3% among the organic crops, and far higher among the commercially grown crops. He and many other pioneers of agriculture and organic farming, such as Lady Even Balfour, one of the founding members of the British Soil Association showed very clearly that the micro-organisms in the soil are the unpaid workers responsible for producing healthy plant life in any soil. Anything that damages or creates imbalances in the micro-organism populations in the soil will result in a relative loss of nutrient density and overall quality in the plants grown therein.

The plants we eat not only depend on healthy soil, which can't possibly occur when being drenched in very dangerous pesticides and chemical fertilizers, *but the animals depend on healthy plants to eat as well.* If you damage the soil, you damage everything that grows in it. Since most of the animals we eat, eat plants; we are foolish to believe that we can have healthy animals when they are being fed very poor quality foods. Much of what commercial farmers feed commercially raised farm animals are grains that have been rejected for use in the human food chain due to dangerously high levels of *mycotoxins.* Mycotoxins are toxins produced by funguses that infect crops that have low levels of vitality. Mycotoxins are some of the most deadly poisons every found. So deadly in fact, that they are used in the biological warfare industry!

The other thing we must remember is that animals are *bio-accumulators.* This means that animals concentrate both nutrition and toxins in their bodies; the bigger the animal the greater the degree of bio-accumulation. In general, researchers have suggested that it takes about six pounds of plant food to create one pound of animal flesh. If you consider the toxins being absorbed by large grazing animals like cows, and add to that the huge amount of drugs and other negative environmental influences the animals are exposed to, it becomes easy to see why *cheap food isn't so cheap after all!*

As we come around the *Wheel of Life,* we find that man's existence is entirely dependent upon the previous links in what could rightly be described as *the chain of life.* In this regard, Sir Albert Howard said,

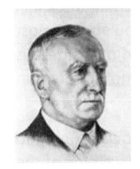

"The birthright of all living things is health. This law is true for soil, plant, animal and man: the health of these four is one connected chain. Any weakness or defect in the health of any earlier link in the chain is carried on to the next and succeeding links, until it reaches the last, namely man."

We humans are at the top of the food chain, but can we really afford to be ignorant, or disrespectful to all the animals, plants and soil micro-organisms that underpin, literally create the foundation of life as we know it? Are we really saving any money by buying cheap food at large chain stores selling the foods created in large factory farming environments?

When "Cheap" Becomes Expensive!

Healthcare costs for American families in 2012 **exceeded $20,000 for the first time**. The annual Milliman Medical Index (MMI) measures the total cost of healthcare for a typical family of four covered by a preferred provider organization (PPO) plan. The 2012 MMI cost is $20,728, an increase of $1,335, or 6.9% over 2011. The rate of increase is not as high as in the past, but the total dollar increase was still a record. This is the first year the average cost of healthcare for the typical American family of four has surpassed $20,000.

Regardless of where you live, the medical costs individually or per family are relatively the same. Yes, there are countries with socialized medicine like Canada and Sweden, but you are the ones constantly facing tax increases to cover these costs. In the end, *there are no free lunches!*

Therefore, the $20,000 question is… *how much organic, free-range, whole foods could you buy for $20,000?* As Jo Rushton points out in this book, *you are what you eat!*

ENS CONTROL RELATIONSHIPS

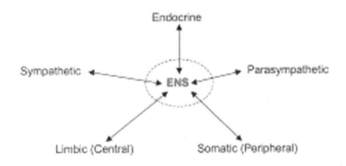

The enteric nervous system (ENS) is more commonly known as the *solar plexus*. The solar plexus is a massive nerve complex with more neurons than your entire brain and spinal cord combined. In my diagram above, you can see the letters "ENS" surrounded by a dotted circle. That dotted circle represents your small intestine, where you absorb most of your food and nutrients. It is also where you absorb most of the dangerous farming chemicals and drugs, as well as the myriad of dangerous food additives, preservatives, colourings, emulsifiers and stabilizers, not to mention the many chemicals from packaging the leach into your foods.

Please take special note of the fact that there are double-ended arrows running *to and from* the lumen of the small intestine and the essential control systems of the human body. "Endocrine" is a medical word for "hormone", and therefore, denotes your hormonal system at large.

Next, on the left you see the word "Sympathetic" and to the right you see the word "Parasympathetic". These are the two branches of your autonomic nervous system (ANS). The ANS is responsible for regulating almost every function in your body aside from your conscious choices. Your ANS regulates your heart and circulation, breathing, digestion, elimination, hormonal functions, metabolism, assimilation, the focus of your eyes, the tone of your muscles, your body temperature, and much more!

Below and to the left, you see the word "Limbic". The limbic system is a complex integration of subsystems in your brain and is responsible for your ability to experience emotion; *pain is technically an emotion by the way.* It is a chief player in your "sentience"; your ability to sense and know yourself as you. It is involved in all mental-emotional disorders as well as any and all experiences perceived as painful, joyous, or otherwise. It is recognized as being integral to your capacity to create, and sense *well-being.*

Below to the right, you see the word "Somatic", which means "of the body". Your body tissues, skin, muscles, the stuff your body is made of, are all "soma".

The essential message from this diagram that I'd love you to understand before you have to learn about it as a patient in some clinic or hospital, is that the food you eat has a direct influence on every one of these major control systems and functions of your body. This is exactly why Hippocrates informed us that *food should be man's first medicine.*

If you could get a rebate for all the money you've spent in your life seeking medical help and using drugs to address the dysfunction created in these systems from cheap food alone, most all of you could certainly afford certified organic food! If you consider the environmental impacts and costs from commercially farmed plants and animals, commercial food is dangerously expensive. Some of the chemicals used in commercial farming take extremely long to break down; guaranteeing that the environment you leave behind by participating in this scam *will be your children's inheritance*. I think they deserve better, don't you?

You Are Rechargeable!

We are living bio-batteries. Just as you need electricity to recharge the battery in your phone, food is a major contributor to recharging your body-mind. The food we eat is not just about molecules that are processed as chemicals in our body to be burnt like fuel in a car engine. Foods bring in light and release light into our body-mind. Haven't you ever eaten something fresh and raw, like a juicy apple and felt a surge of energy before you'd even finished the first bite or two?

Well, considering that the energy from such foods could never be absorbed in less than about twenty minutes for fruit and 3-5 hours for most flesh foods, you have to ask, where did all that energy come from? The answer is simply *light emission*. Your whole energy field, you aura, is made of light. There are many high-tech camera systems used in medical diagnostics today that take pictures of your energy field, and can photograph the energy fields on foods too.

When you have been in a dark room for too long and feel dull, how long does it take before you begin to feel better when you walk out into the sunlight? Not long. All our foods are made of light, and build their bodies out of light. When foods are unhealthy, the light emitted from them is weak and the patterns of energy emitted are dissonant, chaotic. When foods are organic, they emit much more light energy and the patterns emitted from them are more harmonious, nourishing our body immediately. If you want to learn more about this, do a Google search of the keyword "biophoton emission". Look for the works of *Fritz Albert Popp*. You will find others showing these things as well.

Fortunately for me, I don't need to rely on science to tell me these things because I can see and feel the energy fields emanating from all things, living and seemingly inert. Many ask me how I acquired this ability. I tell them that one of the most essential things you can do to reach your human potential is to love and care for yourself. *That includes eating the highest quality foods you possibly can.* That also includes drinking the best quality of water you can get or create with filtration and energizing systems. The next thing I tell them is that when you learn to love and nurture Mother Nature, *she undresses for you and reveals some of her many secrets!* Believe me; she puts on quite a show. Star Wars and Batman are lame in comparison. If you don't believe me, *go look in the mirror!*

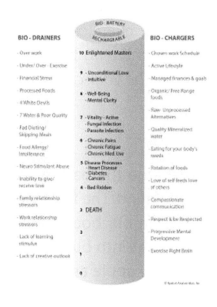

In the bio-battery diagram, you can see that if your overall level of vitality drops below 7 out of 10, you are susceptible to fungal and parasite infections. Currently, there are a number of estimates suggesting that about 90% of the people in the world suffer from both. As your life-force energy diminishes, you can see what kind of common problems emerge.

It is essential to remember that food is one of your primary sources of both nutrition and energy. It is also worth remembering that if the food you are eating is *more dead than you are, you will have to use your own energy to convert it into energy and human tissues.* Most people don't realize that much of their consumption of coffee, stimulants in general, and high-sugar fast foods, is driven by the fact that they keep eating energy deficient, dead foods. Add the chemicals and plastics that end up in foods and you've got the cost of trying to perpetually detoxify yourself.

Looking along the left hand column under "Bio-drainers", it is important to realize that the foods people eat are either directly or indirectly involved in every one of them. Using your mouth as a garbage can is obviously a direct influence. Realizing that the function of your mind and sense of self is heavily influenced by the foods you eat means that all aspects of your stress perception are influenced by what you eat and drink. Quite simply, if there is one thing you can do for yourself that is SURE to speed healing and minimize the risk of fatigue, illness and disease, *it is to eat good food!*

References:

Howard, Sir Albert. (1972). *An Agricultural Testament.* Rodale Press.

2. 2012 Milliman Medical Index. 15 May, 2012. Available from: http://insight.milliman.com/article.php?cntid=8078

THE END

ACKNOWLEDGEMENTS

There are many people who have contributed to ROCKET FUEL ON A BUDGET, some unknowingly and some directly; yet every one of them has been pivotal in my personal growth and development as a human being. Their teachings, support, encouragement, friendship, love and understanding has been the ingredient that has allowed me to embrace all that I am today and to stay true to doing what I love.

My deepest gratitude to:

Pam and Steve Brossman, a powerful duo that have provided me with the structure and the 'know-how' for self-publishing my first book.

My teachers and mentors; Paul Chek, In'Easa Mabulshtar, Qala Sriama, Phoenix, Vidya McNeil and Donal Carr.

Photographer Helen Coetzee, for her friendship, amazing eye and spontaneous creative nature. Working with you was so easy, fun and you made it a breeze!

My dear friends that have supported me throughout the creative process, often witnessing me pull my hair out over writing meal plans and recipes! Fiona Pascoe, Emma Cruikshank, Jesper Lowgren, Caro Webster – thank you all.

The two beautiful little men in my life, my step sons, Oliver and Phoenix Pascoe, for their continual support and questioning "have you finished your book yet, Jo?" This book is one that I trust will support them in their growth and development to the incredible, creative, adults they are on their way to become.

Lastly and most importantly, my wonderful partner, whose loving words of encouragement and copious cups of herbal tea kept the creativity flowing. Thank you for all your help and for coordinating ALL the behind-the-scene activities that helped to bring this book to life.

Thank you.

My thanks to you, the reader, for caring enough about yourself to delve into a book of this nature.

I am the Founder of the Energy Coaching Institute and I am also an internationally qualified chef, exercise and energy specialist. I look forward to supporting you in reclaiming your life force in order to reach your highest personal and professional potential. I trust that this book will support you to your next level of health and wellness. Take care of yourself.

Please visit my website www.energycoachinginstitute.com/rocket-fuel-on-a-budget/ to find out more about me as well as the services we provide.

If you'd like to connect regarding the services I provide or to order copies of this book, it's easy to connect, you can drop me a line on email; jo@energycoachinginstitute.com or phone me on +61 412 271 224.

I look forward to speaking with you and to identifying how we can together create a strategy to increase energy and vitality in your life.

Yours in vibrant health, Jo Rushton

Index & References

Breakfasts:

Lunches:

SMART Analogy
See *7. Relying on discipline alone to reach your goals Pg. 4*

Soy
See *Myths and Truths Pg. 8*

REFERENCES

(1) Paul Chek Author of How To Eat Move And Be Healthy Pg. v, vii, 131, 139-144

(2) Deborah Woodhouse author of Out smarting The Female Fat Cell Pg. 3

(3) Monsanto Co GMO foods Pg. 7

(4) David Getoff's Food Pyramid Pg. 7

(5) Bruce Lipton author of Biology of Belief Pg. 8

(6) Dr Weston A Price author of Nutrition and Physical Degeneration Pg. 11

(7) Dr Malcolm Kendrick author of The great Cholesterol Con Pg. 12

(8) Nora Gedgaudas author of Primal Mind, Primal Body Pg. 12

(9) The work of Uffe Ravnskov MD phD Pg. 12

(10) World Wildlife Foundation (WWF) Pg. 112

(11) Dr Weston A Price author of Nutrition and Physical Degeneration Pg. 112

(12) Professor Seralini Pg. 113

(13) Monsanto Co Pg. 113

(14) Wall Street Journal Pg. 114

(15) Jeffery M Smith Director of Genetic Roulette, the dangers of GMO foods Pg. 114

(16) (WWF) Pg. 114

(17) Dr Candice Peart author of Molecules of Emotion Pg. 114

(18) Food Inc Pg. 114

(19) Sweet Misery Pg. 114

(20) The Cure Pg. 114

(21) Food Matters Pg. 114

(22) Hungry 4 Change Pg. 114

(23) Heart Foundation Pg. 114

(24) Rudolph Steiner Pg. 118

(25) The Organic Certification Directory Pg. 119

(26) The Environmental Working Group (EWG) Pg. 125

(27) Deborah Woodhouse author of Out smarting The Female Fat Cell Pg. 128

(28) Dr Batmangheildj author of Your Body's Many Cries for Water Pg. 130

(29) Paul Chek principles of working In Pg. 131

(30) Doug Kaufmann author of The Fungal Link Pg. 131

(31) Houghton Mifflin author of How The New Science Of Gratitude Can Make You Happier Pg. 131

(32) Bruce Lipton author of Biology of Belief   Pg. 132

(33) Robert Emmons author of Thanks Pg. 132

(34) World Health Organisation Pg. 113

ABOUT THE AUTHOR

Joanna Rushton is an internationally qualified chef, exercise and energy specialist. She's a highly sought after presenter, facilitator, energy coach and holistic chef, working in corporate and health and wellness industries.

She regularly consults to corporate wellness companies, designing proactive resilience programs for executives, and is considered an authority on best practices for building personal health and resilience in the workplace.

Jo delights in sharing the latest research that confronts a decade of misleading health and dietary guidelines. She eloquently debunks the myths that keep us from the real truth that underpins optimal and sustainable energy levels, keeping organisations and their people operating at their fullest potential.

Throughout her 12 years as a chef working in Europe, America, South Africa and Australia, Jo has developed a deep appreciation for whole organic foods and their innate life force.

Her career in the integrative health industry began over ten years ago from her time as a personal trainer and competitive body builder.

"The experience gained as a body builder taught me everything I needed to know about how *not* to train and fuel the body!" She states.

Her passion led her to become a registered CHEK Exercise Coach & Holistic Lifestyle Coach, Level 3. Today she specialises in corrective exercise, rehabilitation and holistic health and lifestyle planning.

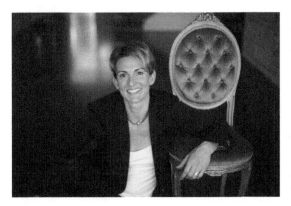

Jo's dedication and commitment to the CHEK approach has led her to become an Assistant Member of C.H.E.K Faculty where she teaches HLC Level 1 Australia-wide and in New Zealand.

Jo Rushton is the CEO and Founder of the Energy Coaching Institute. For further information visit www.energycoachinginstitute.com

CONNECT WITH JO ONLINE:

Facebook: Profile: http://www.facebook.com/joanna.rushton.5
Page: http://www.facebook.com/pages/Energy-Coaching-
Institute/113451455466483

LinkedIn: http://au.linkedin.com/pub/joanna-rushton/3a/3b4/1a2

Website: http://www.energycoachinginstitute.com

Did you enjoy this book? Please consider leaving a review on Amazon
http://www.amazon.com/Rocket-Fuel-Budget-Organic-ebook/dp/B00C1SC0KW

Rushton is sharing here, but couldn't do it nearly as elegantly. you must first find a healthy teacher. You've succeeded in w her advice.

Paul Chek, Founder of the C.H.E.K Institute and
PPS Success Mastery Program

CKET FUEL ON A BUDGET' Includes:

cipes
when trying to get healthy and how to avoid them
ng health and vitality to help you get your mojo back
dern day nutritional recommendations

ok and Feel Fantastic While
Organically on a Budget!

f dieting and trying to achieve your optimal weight?

tal fogginess

s bloating or irregular bowel movements?

sting your energy and mental clarity?
ch and every day and start to look younger at the same time?

you!

day is the day to leave your bad eating choices behind
d start feeling and looking better than you have ever felt
fore. Why? Because YOU'RE WORTH IT!

ww.energycoachinginstitute.com

ISBN 978-0-9874915-0-3

90000

9 780987 491503

RRP $29.95

8.50 x 11.00

351

ROCKET FUEL ON A BUDGET

ROC
ON A

How to Ge

JOANNA RUSHTON

CPSIA information can be obtained at www.ICGtesting.com
Printed in the USA
LVOW02s0537190713

343670LV00003B/4/P